TRUTH IN THE DARK

☙ CASEMPIUM Q. JOHNSON ❧

Copyright © 2018 Casempium Q. Johnson
All rights reserved
First Edition

PAGE PUBLISHING, INC.
New York, NY

First originally published by Page Publishing, Inc. 2018

ISBN 978-1-68139-512-8 (Paperback)
ISBN 978-1-68139-513-5 (Digital)

Printed in the United States of America

REMINISCE

How is it possible that I, Jordan Rodgers, find myself right back in my small town of Social Circle, Georgia? Even after a bachelor's degree in business administration, I look at myself, and I'm back in the same old town, more messed up than the day I left. It had been years since I left my hometown of misery and disappointments. Although I was one of the most popular teenagers in high school, I sometimes still felt alone. I never understand how or why trying to be a man can deprive you of discussing your true feelings. Often, as men, we spend so much time trying to showcase to our friends, family members, and people we barely even know that we are masculine. As I sit in my car, thinking, I ask myself, *What makes a man masculine? Why do men feel comfortable displaying their true emotions only in the dark, when there's no one around to comfort them?*

Mary J. Blige plays in the background while I sit in my car. I listen as she soulfully sings, "If you look into my life and see what I see." I continue to think. The fact that I'm sitting alone in my car in my mama's driveway, listening to R&B music by a female, is something I wouldn't do if someone other than my mama was near me. Mary J. Blige is one of my favorite female vocalists, and I listen to her music often but never around my friends. Perhaps society has made me captive of my own emotions, because instead of doing me, I do what I think others will approve of. On second thought, maybe it's just me who holds me a prisoner of my sentiments.

Many times while driving around town in the summer, with humidity thick and the sun shining bright, I would ride in my car, listening to rap music. There were times when I was in a mellow mood and wanted to listen to neo-soul or R&B music while driving with my windows down during the summer. The truth is, my insecurity of being a man wouldn't allow me to. At least that's what I call it—*insecurities*—because if I was really secure with my manhood, I wouldn't care what anyone think about me listening to any kind of music in my own car. Society or maybe just the black community has taught me to hide my deep innermost thoughts if it does not pertain to me being masculine. In other words, the only time I can listen to slow jams is if I have a chick in the car with me. It's funny how the dumpiest shit would make the fellows question your sexuality. Growing up in a small town has its ups and downs. Most of the people living here, including my peers and the elderly, are not open-minded. The slightest thing that a young man or woman did different is questionable to everyone in my hometown.

When I was a junior in high school, I convinced Quinesha to let a couple of my friends take turns having sex with her. My home boys as well as many other boys that knew her would call her a freak because of how easy she was to give up some pussy.

My homies Fred and Markus were excited about the adventures with Quinesha. I wasn't thrilled or turned up about the situation because I had already dived in the deepest part of her ocean a few times, so I was passing her on to my friends.

"Y'all niggas can smash first. I had her last week, so I might just pass on getting some ass from her tonight," I said.

"Thanks, bruh! How was it, man? Was it wet like a river?" said Fred with a big grin on his face.

Fred was six foot three and used to getting pleasure from some of the finest girls near him, because the ladies seem to love a man who's tall. That's why I'm happy to be five foot eleven and knocking on the door of being taller than six feet. Unfortunately, my growth spurt has deserted me, but trust me, I still have no problem getting the ladies. With my athletic build, my 360 waves, and my charisma, I could have most girls eating out my hand.

As if I were thinking out loud, I smiled and told Fred, "Trust me, homey, it's wetter than the ocean, damn a river, and you know an ocean is deep." As we both laughed, I told him, "So get ready to dive in, but don't drown in it."

"She easy and a quick fuck, so I'm going treat that hoe like she present herself and pass her to the next man in line after I'm done with her." Fred then turned and looked at Markus with a smirk. "Aye yo! Markus, you ready to lose your virginity?"

"I never said I was a virgin. Just because I don't kiss and tell or fuck and tell don't mean I'm a virgin. Chill!" Markus quickly replied.

"If you ain't a virgin, tell me why you getting all offensive when clearly I'm just joking with you? So calm down, boy," said Fred.

"Both of y'all, calm down, because there's no need to mess up your friendship over a girl who probably will hook up with anything who has something hard between their legs," I said.

I remember that night well because it was one of the few times that Quinesha would get the crib all too herself. Her parents were both churchgoing people and were very strict on Quinesha, especially her dad. Somehow she would always seem to find a way to sneak out to hook up with boys. Even though her dad was meaner than the devil, Quinesha would risk getting chastised by her dad for that prized possession that boys had between their legs. I guess what they say is true about a PK (preacher kid), that they are usually freaks to the core. Quinesha was a living example of that, but I would be lying if I said I never ponder why a PK would turn out so promiscuous.

"Fred, you go first while Markus and I be your lookout. Her window is on the left side of the house, so we will park near the curve close to the stop sign so we can not only watch for you but inform you if her parents' Cadillac pulls up. If we blow the horn, that means run your ass out and hop in the car so we can go," I said.

"A'ight, that's a bet," Fred said as he checked his pocket for a condom.

Quinesha lived in a subdivision with a plethora of stop signs and sidewalks, and her house was the first one on the left once you passed three stops signs. The fact that there were three stop signs to go through before her parents reached their house and it was dark outside was an advantage for us. Quinesha's parents seemed to be smart people, so I never understood how they could be so naive when it came to their daughter. Quinesha was a Georgia peach and was thicker than grits with a body that screamed voluptuous. In fact, if any man didn't know what the word meant, all he had to do was look at her and he would quickly comprehend the definition of *voluptuous*. The only imperfection she had was, occasionally her right eye would wander, causing her to have a lazy eye. I'm not sure why a girl as fine as her would put herself out like that. Maybe it's wrong of me to allow a young black woman to violate her body like that, but then again, she was having sex with various boys at her own discretion. She wouldn't even care about what people said about her behind her back, or at least it didn't seem to faze her. No matter how many girls talked down about her and ridicule her name, she still continued to do what made her happy. It just seemed that sleeping with boys made her happy. In some ways, I wish I had the courage to go against the grain and do what makes me happy. No one can live my life for me or walk in my shoes, right? Markus interrupted my thoughts with a burst of excitement, and I turned to him with a puzzled look.

"Aye! That's my shit, Jay, turn that up," Markus said as he started nodding his head to the music and pumping himself up.

I turned the volume up on the radio without hesitation, as I too started nodding my head to the song, and in unison, we sang the lyrics to one of our favorite rap songs. "To the window, to the wall, to sweat drip down my…" We both rapped as we enjoyed the music of Lil Jon and the Ying Yang Twins' classic dirty south song.

"I haven't heard this song in long-ass time, bruh," Markus said loudly over the music. "It brings back memories!"

"Markus, I see Fred on his way back to the car, you up next. You have a rubber on you?"

"Yeah, I made sure that I keep one in my wallet at all times. I'm not ready to be a dad, especially not to someone I don't love or have feelings for."

"I hear you, but shut up with all that mushy stuff." As we both laughed, Fred had made it back to the car, boasting about how he wore her out. As I watched Markus get out the front seat and Fred slide in the front seat, I still was staying alert. Nothing would distract me from keeping a solid lookout for Quinesha's parents' car as I studied every car that pulled up at the first stop sign in her subdivision. Fred had calmed down from bragging about the sexual positions he had Quinesha do and how he had her moaning long enough for me to listen to the radio and think. Looking at Markus walk up to the house made me smile to myself because I remembered that he's shorter than the girl that waited for him in the house. Quinesha was a five-foot-nine pecan-brown queen, or should I say, sex queen, while Markus on the other hand stood at five foot seven. Although Markus was short, he's no one's punk and was built like a college football player. He took pride in his physique. Since he had been introduced to weight training in middle school, he's been going steady at lifting weights. I've heard plenty of girls say, "His strength makes up for his height."

After about fifteen minutes, he came back to the car with a stern look on his face, like he was deep in thought. Fred didn't seem to notice, but since he was asleep as if he was the one worn out instead of Quinesha, I didn't expect him to notice Markus's return. Besides the radio playing, we drove off in silence, not saying a word to each other. I knew something was wrong, so I didn't want to press Markus about it at the moment. Although, I was extremely curious about what was the matter with my best friend.

A few days went by and I had heard a rumor with Markus's name in it, which I didn't believe for one minute. A few people were saying that Quinesha was telling people that Markus was gay. She went on to inform people that when she and Markus tried to be intimate, he couldn't get it up, so that must mean one thing…that he's gay. When Markus found out he, became furious and almost punched Quinesha when confronting her during our lunch break at school. If I wasn't there, he probably would have hit her in front of a school full of witnesses. After managing to make our way through the circle of students watching the dispute like movie at the matinee, we went outside to talk alone.

"Markus, what's your problem!" I screamed out of shock, not anger. "Don't you know that you could get in serious trouble for putting your hands on a girl?"

"Fuck that, Jay!" Markus screamed, matching the amplitude of my voice with the anger of his own. "She got people questioning if I'm a faggot! I'm not like other niggas in this school who brag about how many women they sleep with to make their self look like a king of all kings."

"I feel ya. Aye, man, you can talk to me about what really happened. I'm listening. I know you straight, and I won't judge you."

"Once I got in the room with Quinesha, I just didn't feel right about the situation. I mean, usually I'm dating a girl and getting to know her before having sex with her. My parents always taught me to respect a woman even if she doesn't respect herself. Every day I try to live by those words and apply it to my life. The fact that I never had sex with a woman that I never dated made it difficult to get aroused, so I had to stay true to myself. That's when I walked out of the room and came back to the car that night so we can leave."

"I think I understand what you saying. But how you going to live by your parents' principles and respect a woman if you hit a woman?"

"I never hit a woman before, but a woman never talked so poorly about me before. I need to do some soul-searching and make sure I never come close to hitting a woman again."

In that moment, I understood Markus and respected him even more because he was able to admit when he's wrong. Not only did he admit when he's wrong, but he stood up for what he believed in by not sleeping with Quinesha. The situation got me to thinking. How is it that when you question men's sexuality, they become violent or livid? I'm sure I would be able to tell if someone, especially a man, is gay. Most gay men usually fit a stereotype, and none of my friends fits any of those stereotypes. I would know when someone is homosexual, whether it's a man or a woman.

Snapping out of my memories that plague my mind of the past, I realize that I didn't know a gay man if he stood right in front of me. If I did, I can't help to think that my life would remain the same, but instead, the view of things in my life has changed.

GRADUATION

The sky was clear and blue while the sun was beaming radiantly on my head. I couldn't help but think, *Damn, I will be glad when this ceremony is over. It's hot as fuck in Atlanta today.* The clouds seemed to be dancing around the sun today, as oppose to dancing in front of the sun. This was supposed to be one of the happiest days of my life, graduating from Clark Atlanta University with a 3.5 GPA and earning my bachelor's degree in business administration. If the truth be told, I wasn't as happy as I should be. I had no clue if Markus's and my future plans after college would come through for us or fall apart. Looking around the field as I look at some of my fellow classmates dressed in black and red caps and gowns, I was certain that I wasn't the only one unsure about what the future holds for a college graduate. Some of the other people had the same look on their face as I did. Our expression read that we were ready to get this shit over with so we can move on with our life. Just in the nick of time, I heard someone calling my name.

"Jordan Miles Rodgers earned a bachelor's degree in business administration with a GPA of 3.5," Mr. Brown said with a smile of approval for me to make my way to the podium. I started to make my way to the podium and was quite thankful that one of my favorite professors was giving out our degree certificates. Before I could make my way to the podium, out the corner of my eye, I saw a proud mama snapping pictures of me. I knew then that it had to be my own mama documenting this memorable moment through photos. Before I could look her way for a quick picture, Mrs. Cheryl Rodgers shouted out, "That's my boy!" I was slightly embarrassed, but I put aside those feelings away, because after all, I knew she loved me. She was proud of me.

After what seemed like a long draining day in the heat, the ceremony was about over. The indication of everyone throwing their caps up in the air was the traditional way of ending the ceremony. Soon after, everyone and their mamas would find the college graduate they knew, and they would congregate with each other. With open arms, my mama came rushing toward me like a pro football player playing defense in a Super Bowl game.

"Baby, I'm so proud of you!" she said with excitement and with tears in her eyes.

"I know, Mama, and I saw you snapping pictures like you're a photographer. I hope you got my good side, or I will consider firing you," I said while we shared a laugh and embraced each other like a close mother and son would.

"I carried you for nine months, so there ain't any firing or replacing me."

"I know! I know!" I said jokingly and looked around. "Where is everyone else?"

"They went back to your Uncle Joe's house in East Point to finish setting up for our party, or should I say family gathering?" With her hands on her hips, she continued and said, "Lord knows I still got the moves, so I might show a few of my party girl moves at the family celebration."

I just looked at my mama and all her sassiness and just smiled. My mama is forty-two years old. She had me when she was my age of twenty-one. Now standing at five foot six and still petite with sandy-brown skin that's flawless, my mama didn't look like she was past the age of thirty. Women would envy her because of her swagger and the attention she would get when she walks into a room. Not only the way she looks was angelic, but the way she carried herself was angelic as well. Very few women befriended her. The few that did were usually true friends, because the other women were so jealous of her beauty that they couldn't stand to speak to her. This is how the women treat her now, since I've been old enough to remember her, and only God knows how they treated her before I was born.

Single and married men tried to take my mama out on dates, but she would shut them down. For some odd reason, she was devoted to a man that I barely knew and whom I was told could be my twin. Samuel Rodgers, or who people say is my twin, is my father, but he was never there for me like I needed him to be. He was always in and out our lives whenever he pleased. My mama loved him deeply. She loved him so unconditionally that she's still married to him after twenty-two years. He left us when I was still in my mother's womb because he was afraid of the responsibility. When I thought of him, I began to sternly clinch my teeth together without knowing it.

On cue, my mama noticed and said, "I know that look because that's the same look your dad would give when something is bothering him. So tell me what's wrong."

"Nothing major," I said without looking into her eyes.

"I'm sure I know why you have that look on your face. I won't say any names, but Jordan, baby…he loves you even though he doesn't show it at times. I've known him for over twenty years. He's just hurting from making a decision that he thought was so right years ago. Y'all have got to forgive each other."

"If he cares so much, why isn't he here? Why did he walk out on us before I was born?"

"He isn't here because he knew if he did, it would upset you. He didn't want you to become furious on a day that you should be overwhelmed with joy. We can finish talking about this later, so don't think about it anymore today. I want you to enjoy your day and your night."

"Okay," I said as I gave my mama another hug.

After one final embrace and reminder to meet the family at my Uncle Joe's house in an hour and half, she then dashed off to prepare for the family dinner. Almost immediately after my mama left, my best friend, Markus, greeted me with a congratulation for our accomplishments. That's been my right-hand man since high school when he moved from South Georgia with his parents. Now we both were college educated, with plans to become business partners. Two brothers who beat the odds of being a menace to society with the privilege of earning a degree—this moment is priceless. Our dream is to open up a sports bar called Gear Up Sports Bar & Grill. After starting a successful bar and grill, we want to invest in starting a sports store with the same name. Hell yeah, we were some ambitious mothafuckas who have big dreams. After dabbing each other hands with a manly half hug, we separated before Markus said to me with a huge grin, "We did it! We some damn college graduates." With such a joyful expression written all over his face, I knew Markus was proud of our accomplishment.

"Yup! You better know it, because we did the damn thang!" I said with a tone of excitement.

"Have you spoken to Fred?"

"Matter a fact, I did this morning before I left my dorm. He said he won't make the graduation, but he's coming to the graduation party tonight."

"He should've been on the field with us, receiving a certificate of some kind. He's smarter than what he makes his self seem."

"I totally agree with you, but he's convinced that working at some factory is the career path he wants. We tried to dispute the idea by telling him that there's money to be made out here than to be hitting the time clock in a factory all your life."

"Yeah, man, it seems like he's caught up in living that country-ass lifestyle instead of trying to live the good life," Markus said, shaking his head in disbelief as he continued, "At least he's a man standing on his own two feet. I can say that he's independent and making grown decisions for himself, as opposed to being peer pressured into doing something someone else wants him to do. I still wish he would change his mind about becoming business partners with us."

"Yeah, man. Together all three of us could be like the friends who started Facebook. Now they make billions of dollars off an idea."

I noticed Markus's eyes drifted to the left of me. He smiled while licking his lips seductively, so I followed his gaze. There she was, a five-foot-five golden-light-skinned girl with deep dimples that left an imprint on her face even when she wasn't smiling. Asia, with a signature stylish short haircut, was walking toward Markus with the same seductive look in her eyes. Asia and Markus dated through their four years of college. The two of them were now engaged and planned to get married soon. Markus was a man of integrity. If he believed in something, he stood by it no matter what, and he believed that Asia was the girl of his dreams, so he proposed to her a week before graduation. In some ways I wish I could learn to please myself more often than please everyone else. I believe someone who does what makes them happy is truly a leader, not a follower.

With a big smile, Asia said to me, "Congratulations!" and then she reached out to give me a hug before I could say thank you and congratulate her. Markus grabbed her from behind with a kiss on her neck. As I said my congrats, she turned around to greet her fiancée with a wet kiss that lasted for like hours. Those two had no problem with showing public affection for each other. They didn't give a damn who saw them holding hands or kissing. I looked away for a moment instead of watching the freak show they were displaying. I looked around to see if I saw my girlfriend, Destiny, among the plethora of people. I knew she would be somewhere near because this was her graduation too.

Breaking me out my search for my girlfriend, Asia said, "You looking for Destiny? She said she spotted you and told me to tell you that she will be over in a few."

With a surprised look and smile, I said, "You read my mind. I'm going make sure I tell everyone to call you, you know, for their free psychic reading." We all laughed.

"Shut up, punk, don't get all dramatic on me," Asia teased.

"What time is Destiny's party?" Markus said.

"It starts at ten tonight," I said.

"Speaking of Destiny, there she goes right behind you."

Right on cue, I felt some small arms around my waist holding on to me. Even if Markus didn't tell me she was behind me, I would've known who it was because of the scent of her perfume. She liked to mix her perfume with Bath & Body Works products to carry a scent that no one else has. It's a scent that I was very familiar with. Destiny lived up to her name; she's my fortune, a rear jewel that only the fortunate will discover, and I was so blessed that she's my treasure. In a world where most black men go for the lighter skin complexion, I was completely satisfied with the dark-chocolate skin tone of my queen.

All four of us chatted some more about our short- and long-term goals as well as how far we came before promising that we will meet up at the party again for more celebration. Now that I was off to meet up with my family for our gathering, I couldn't help to think that a year has gone by since Destiny and I'd been dating, so I think it's time to tell her how I feel about our relationship tonight. I just wanted to make sure that she understands that I love her. We also needed to talk about our future together after college, because most of past and present has been built around college. I assumed that conversation can wait, because we have some celebrating to do, starting with my family.

FAMILY CELEBRATION

Instead of going to my dorm and changing clothes, I thought it would be best if I took some changing clothes with me. Since most of my relatives didn't take pictures with me right after graduation, I was sure they will at the family gathering. With that in mind, I made sure I left my cap and gown in the car for additional pictures with my family in my honorable uniform. Looking in the mirror, I checked myself to make sure my black slacks and black-and-red pin-striped short-sleeved dress shirt were still looking perfect. I thought to myself, *Thank you, God, for blessing me with sex appeal and good looks*. I chuckled to myself after a final look over in the mirror before I adjusted my red silk tie, then I was on my way out the door.

As I pulled up to my Uncle Joe's highly black-populated neighborhood in East Point, Georgia, I saw many of my relatives' automobiles. It didn't take long for me to find a parking spot. My uncle Joe was so generous. He saved a parking spot for me in his driveway. The sign he placed at the end of his driveway behind his cars stated, "This parking spot is saved for my nephew only." That made me feel special. It looked like this family gathering was shaping up to be a nice family affair after all. Although I didn't have any doubt it wouldn't be, because my mama's side of the family always knew how to party. My family loved to see everyone having a great time, so she invited some of my dad's family over too. I usually called him Samuel since he played the dad role so poorly. Samuel's family declined and made up alibis on why they couldn't come, which didn't surprise me. They hardly ever had family gatherings. They were the complete opposite of my mama's family. I can at least say that most of Samuel's family reached out to me to tell me how proud they were of my major accomplishment.

In all honesty, the one Rodger I hoped don't call me today was my dad. I suppose the fact that my dad didn't have a close connection with his own father was maybe the reason why there's a lack of unity between him and me. Could it be that he had an absent father figure in his life, causing him the inability to love his only son? Perhaps if he wasn't raised in a single-parent home, he would know how to cherish his wife and most importantly his only son.

As I parked and turned off the ignition, I saw my nieces and nephews playing all the fun games I used to play when I was their age: Mother, may I, Simon says, as well as freeze tag. Childhood memories sometimes made me smile even without having a stable male figure in my life. After I placed the ignition to rest, I gathered up my belongings to join everyone in the backyard. Not another second, minute, or hour longer did I want to miss out on all the fun, so I quickly grabbed my stuff out the backseat to join everyone. With my keys in my left hand, I put my cap and gown back on to make my entrance toward the backyard.

The grill was fired up, sending the aroma of baby back ribs, hamburgers, hot dogs, and barbeque chicken floating in the summer breeze. I closed my eyes to imagine. *This must be what heaven smells like.* After a few seconds of smelling heaven in the evening, I opened my eyes and said out loud with big grin, "Barbeque food has never smelt better." My mouth was watering for a nice well-done juicy cheeseburger, baked beans, and some spicy-flavored SunChips. As I entered the backyard, everyone noticed. My family, along with some family friends, had me feeling like I was an Oscar-winning actor stepping out on the red carpet. Everyone wanted a picture, a hug, or a handshake from me. After the picture taking, I took my cap and gown off for good this time.

"Hey, my man! Nephew, I'm proud of you, boy," Uncle Joe said as he approached me from the grill. "I left the steak I'm going to cook for you in the fridge. It's been marinating overnight. I'm about to get ready to place that bad boy on the grill."

Uncle Joe has always looked out for me. I respected him. He was the father figure I never had, besides my mama playing the role of my mother and father.

"Thanks, Unk! And I can tell someone's been eating too many steaks on and off the grill," I said as I teased my Uncle Joe.

"Hold up now, nephew. This old man might've packed on some weight since my younger days, but trust me, this old man will still kick your ass," Uncle Joe said as he playful punched me in my stomach. He stood there in this apron in his boxing stance, like he was Muhammad Ali fighting for the championship belt. I pretended like I was afraid of him and grimaced in pain like I was hurt.

"No need to beat me up. This man knows how to back down." We both laughed as he lowered his hands and hugged me.

"I love you, nephew, just like you're my own son."

"I know, Unk. I love you as well."

"Tell my baby sis to bring me the steak out the fridge so I can cook it for you. She's in the kitchen with Beverly."

"Okay, will do," I said as I turned around to walk toward the patio door that was not far from the family-size pool.

Everyone seemed to be having a great time listening to music and chatting while waiting for the food to finish cooking on the grill. There were some of my family playing cards about fifty feet between the patio and the pool. Four of my family members were playing spades, talking shit, and drinking beer. The teenagers were playing dice, swimming, playing basketball, or playing pool inside. When I finished delivering my uncle's message, I planned on returning back outside where almost everyone was to fellowship with my beloved family that I cherish so much.

Once I made it in the kitchen, Beverly was the first person I noticed wearing her favorite color, pink. Beverly is my Uncle Joe's wife. She had on a pink and white tank top shirt with beige shorts and thong sandals. She was a very voluptuous woman with curves in all the right places. My uncle was truly a lucky man.

"Oh! Cheryl, look what the cat brought in," Beverly said with so much excitement I thought she caught the Holy Ghost.

I couldn't stop myself from chuckling softly. In a swift move, my mama dropped what she was doing and looked up at me with a smile of delightfulness. Next to Beverly was my mom wearing a blue apron over her yellow sundress, with her hair pulled back in a ponytail.

My mama picked back up the mixing bowl and said, "I'm glad you made it, son. I'm almost done fixing your favorite dessert. I wanted to surprise you, but you caught me red-handed in here baking you some sweets."

She knew that I haven't had a caramel cheesecake since Christmas when I was back home visiting her for the holiday season. I couldn't wait until I tasted the first bite. My mama was good at baking. That was something she did exceptionally well.

"Thanks, Mama. You're the best," I said before I placed a kiss on her cheek.

"Jay, come over here and give your aunt Bev a hug and some suga'," Beverly said. She preferred me to call her Aunt Bev instead of "Yes, ma'am" or "Mrs. Beverly." Before I could give her a hug, she held me in place and said to me, "I was so proud of you graduating today. I just love to see our young black people succeed instead of running the streets trying to be a thug all the damn time."

"I have a strong mother right by myself that wouldn't allow me to get into these streets," I said.

With one hand on her hip, my mama looked at Aunt Bev and then me before saying, "You better know it, because when that ass gets out of line, I had to straighten your ass up."

We all shared a laugh after my mama's comment. She was right; she wouldn't tolerate me getting into trouble or missing up my grades in school. If I did get into trouble, there were serious consequences I had to pay. She would get my own belt to whip me with it.

"Mom, Uncle Joe wants you to bring the T-bone to him now."

With a smirk, my mama said, "You tell that black wannabe Chef Boyardee to come fetch his own food for the rest of the day. Now Bev and I been running food back and forth to him all day."

"Amen!" Bev said with a soft chuckle.

"Hey, just give me the steak. I will take it to him, ladies," I joked back.

In unison, Aunt Bev and my mama, with a smirk on their faces, said, "He tried that!"

We all shared some more laughter before my mama told me where the T-bone was in the fridge so I could take it to my uncle. There was so much good food here that I knew I would eat like a pig. In the kitchen and fridge, I noticed baked beans, a plethora of potato chips, hot dog buns, hamburger buns, potato salad, coleslaw, macaroni and cheese, fried fish, homemade banana pudding, Blue Bell vanilla ice cream, caramel cheesecake, and strawberry short cake. That was only what I saw in the kitchen. There was more good food outside. It was like we had enough food to feed the hungry for a whole year. I couldn't eat everything, so I had to take several to-go plates home. "Thank God I have a high metabolism," I said out loud as I closed the patio door behind me.

Everyone outside seemed to be getting the party turned up, because a *Soul Train* line had formed. The Gap Band song "You Dropped a Bomb on Me" was blasting out the speakers. My uncle even took a break from the grill to get in on some of the action. Old-school music was his favorite. He especially loved the up-tempo old-school songs so he could dance. I could vision him in front and in center on Don Cornelius's syndicated show *Soul Train*, dancing to the latest tunes with his big Afro, along with his platform shoes and bell-bottom pants. Once he got finished dancing down the *Soul Train* line, he went back to the grill to check on the food.

Now I was eager to join the *Soul Train* line, so I jogged over to my uncle to hand him the T-bone then ran over to get in line formation. Anxiously I was waiting for my turn to dance down the *Soul Train* line.

One of my cousins was a successful DJ in Atlanta, so anytime he was free when we needed him to DJ, he would do it free of charge. He was on the turntables now. By time it was my turn to dance down the line, with all eyes on me, he switched it to DJ Unk's "Walk It Out." That used to be my song years ago, so I walked it out, adding my own twist to the hyper dance. I was having so much fun that I wanted to live in this moment forever. Moments like this made me forget about everything. Moments like this made me love being around my family and want to have a family of my own.

"Jay!" I heard someone calling me, waking me up out my trance of joy. I looked where the voice was coming from, only to realize it was my mama calling me from near the end of the *Soul Train* line. I was in my own world I didn't realize she came outside.

"Yes, ma'am?" I said.

"There's someone on the phone for you," she said with a nervous look. In fact, she looked like she wasn't sure if I wanted me to answer the call.

I looked up at her with a confused look, and with concern in my voice, I said, "Who is it?"

She gave me the phone, but the look on her face didn't change. Then she managed to speak and said, "I will allow you to find out for yourself."

I immediately interrupted her and said with curiosity, "But, Mama, why can't you just tell me?"

"Boy, don't you question me. You take this phone and be civil with whomever is on the phone. Do you hear me?" she said with touch of anger that I was questioning her.

I wasn't sure if it was because she thought I was being disrespectful or the fact that I was questioning who was on the phone after she already seemed nervous to give me the phone anyway.

"Yes, ma'am. I hear you," I said then placed the phone to my ear as I watched her walk away back toward the house.

I said hello without looking at the screen on the cell phone. If I did, I probably would've hung up without answering it.

A deep mellow voice that sounded slightly nervous answered and said, "Hello, son. How are you?"

After I heard the voice, I knew exactly who it was—it was Samuel Rodgers. With so much frustration in my voice that I couldn't disguise, I said, "I was doing just fine. What you want?"

"I'm just calling to say hi to my son. I sent you a graduation card in the mail. I know I haven't been there for you in the past, but I'm proud of you, son."

"Okay, I will check my mail when I get to my dorm."

"Jay…I want to let you know that I'm sorry for not being there for you and your mother. Will you forgive me?"

"I will have to think about that, but I have to go, so I will talk to you some other time," I said that in hopes of rushing him off the phone, because I didn't want him to wreck my day thinking about his bullshit lies.

"Okay, son, I will let you do that. Tell your mother that I still love her. And, son, I love you too."

"Yeah, whatever you say man. Bye."

I hung up before he could say anything else to me, shaking my head in disbelief that this dude had the audacity to believe I would forgive him for his impulsive behavior. I didn't believe he loved me or my mama for one second. I just couldn't forget about how he promised me his old Chevrolet Impala on my sixteenth birthday or how many times he promised to spend Father's Day with me but failed to do so. At this point in my life, I was not sure if I should forgive him, but I did know I couldn't forget the shit he didn't do for me. Maybe that's why I couldn't forgive. Maybe I was not over the sadness of not having a full-time father in my life. Just maybe I needed more time to heal… more time to grow.

GRADUATION PARTY

Somehow I managed to not allow the conversation with my distant father to disturb me to the point of no return. Spending time with my family helped lift the weight of my thoughts about my father. The humor of my family also prevented my anguished thoughts from wearing me down. This was my day to celebrate—to be vibrant in my new path in life.

When that family gathering was over, I had to get me a drink. I needed to party a little. I definitely needed to release some stress. That night I needed something or someone to use as my scapegoat. I was twenty-one then. Whether I liked it or not, I was officially an adult. It's time for me to face my life head-on, making my own decisions. I had goals but not sure how to pursue them. I was afraid of failure or being anything like my father more than I was horrified of Freddy Krueger or Jason as a kid.

When I was around ten years old, my Uncle Joe's son, Terrance, dared me to sneak in my mother's room to watch a scary scene from her *Nightmare on Elm Street* DVD.

Terrance said, "I dare you to watch the scariest scene of *Nightmare on Elm Street* by yourself in the dark. Don't be no punk!"

I was so desperate to seem brave and cool at that age that I did almost anything to fit in. Of course, I took the dare head-on like I wasn't petrified about the idea. That same night, I had nightmares of Freddy Krueger chasing me in my dreams. I remember waking up in a cold sweat, not wanting to run to my mother's room but also not wanting to stay in my room alone. Eventually, the nightmares stopped as I made myself realize it wasn't reality. No man with sharp claws can really haunt me in my dreams. The older I became, I recognized what I was truly afraid of. What I was afraid of more than any fictional character or monster was failure. Becoming anything like Samuel Rodgers would be a huge failure to everything I worked hard for. As I stood there that day as an adult, I knew that he's my modern-day Freddy Krueger, who tortured my conscious thoughts daily.

The night was starting to begin. As I looked at my watch, I noticed that it's fifteen minutes past nine p.m. Destiny's party starts at ten until two a.m. An hour ago I had changed into some black shorts, white Polo, and some black-and-red Jays. Since I'd been wearing slacks and a tie all day, I wanted to look casual for my girlfriend's party tonight. I was sure everyone else would dress the same. She was throwing a party with a red, black, and white color theme that matched our school colors. No one was allowed to enter her party if they weren't wearing at least one of those colors.

Destiny was stubborn. When her mind was made up, there was no changing it. After saying good-bye to my family as they left, I received many gifts, hugs, handshakes, and kisses before fixing me a plate to devour for the next couple of days. I got into my car feeling confident that tonight was going to be a good night. Instead of listening to some hip-hop to get turned up before the party, I popped in Mary J. Blige's latest CD, *My Life: The Journey Continues*. At the party, the DJ would play majority of the hottest hip-hop songs, so I figured I would listen to something to help reserve my energy. I turned my AC on and cruised toward I-75 North, toward downtown Atlanta, until I got to Spring Street exit. The party was going to be at Club Primal. Destiny had wealthy parents, so they paid for her to rent out that club tonight for her own private event.

I pulled up at the club, parked my car, and hopped out after placing my Ray-Ban sunglasses on my face. Although there was no sun outside or inside the club, it was a habit of mine to wear shades inside the club. A nice pair of sunglasses gave me the extra confidence I needed to walk like I'm the shit. Walking up to the club past the long line, I went to the VIP line with my swag on a hundred. I felt like I was Atlanta's own Young Jeezy or Ludacris, being able to walk past everyone to get in the club as everyone in the line admired my swag.

Before I could go in, a bouncer stopped me and asked, "Can I see your college ID?" starting at me with a serious look in his eyes. He was tall and brawny like he should be playing for the Atlanta Falcons.

I looked at him without showing any intimidation and said, "I'm Jordan Rodgers. I'm on the VIP list."

He told another guy who was sitting close by who I was. The other guy was shorter than the bouncer I just had a brief chat with. He was about my height but looked like he could be on someone's football field as well. I watched him look over the list in what seemed like seconds before he motioned to the other bouncer to let me through.

The tall club bouncer moved out my way and said, "Al'ight, bruh. You good."

I didn't say anything but just walked past him to meet with the next club bouncer so he could pat me down for weapons. After a quick check for any weapons or anything that the club owner wouldn't allow in his facility, I was itching to get inside. The music was bumping out the speakers, playing Future and Kelly Rowland's hit single. I could imagine that the ladies were getting loose with that song. It seemed like the ladies loved anything that Future puts out, especially down in the dirty south.

The club had a nice-sized crowd, which didn't surprise me. Atlanta had college students all over the city that were partying harder than ever since the summer had begun. Summer meant one thing to college students: party! It was time to put the books and long hours of studying behind for some fun in the nightlife. I knew how sensational it could feel to substitute a book for a drink. There were all types of beautiful women in the club—white, black, Asian, and Latino. Guys weren't just posting up on the wall but were actually trying to dance with the ladies. Everyone in the club seemed to be having a good time.

I walked over toward the bar as I continued to scope the scene of the dance floor, only to notice Markus and Asia walking toward me. I was beside the bar when they approached me, holding hands, with a drink in the other. Both of them looked great together.

With my drink held up high to the sky, doing my two-step to the music, I said, "What up, y'all?"

In unison, both of my friends replied by raising their drinks in the air for a toast as they both said, "What's up?"

Asia had on some black pants, a red sleeveless shirt that stopped a little above her waist, with white accessories, and four-inch black heels. Now she was taller than her fiancée by two inches. Markus had on black Levi jeans with nice loafers and a button-down black-and-red shirt.

"Markus, didn't your ass get tired of a wearing a button-down from being dressed up all day long at graduation?" I said, laughing out loud.

"Nigga, first of all, the graduation didn't last all day long," Markus retaliated.

"I should've known your wannabe old man ass would wear some damn loafers tonight."

"Get off my dick, nigga. I got swag."

Markus wiped off his shoulder as if dust were on it while Asia brushed off the back of his shirt. These two were straight clowning tonight. We all just laughed by the bar, talking and listening to the music. About twenty minutes had gone by, when I noticed Destiny walking toward us from the crowd, dressed in a red, black, and white V-cut shirt with a fitted black skirt. Her hair was well conditioned, looking silky smooth. In that moment, I knew why after a year of dating, I've been devoted only to her. She was my Destiny. She's my princess. I was her prince. Together we could be untouchable. She put the fortune in my fate. With her, I didn't need any good-luck wishes, because she was my lucky star. I loved her.

"Babe, you looking sexy tonight. Damn! If I didn't already have your number, I would ask for it again," I said while looking at her, biting my bottom lip.

Without hesitation, I opened my arms as she wrapped her arms around me. I couldn't wait to feel her body next to mine. The smell of her fragrance was so salacious and sweet. It made me want to kiss her down below. Kelly Rowland ain't the only one who prefers her kisses down low. My baby arches that back for me every time I kiss her below the belt.

"You know I have to look sexy for my boo," Destiny said with a smile.

Asia knocked me out of fantasizing about my girl with a loud greeting. I wasn't mad or surprised, because it's typical for these two to greet each other that way.

"Hey, girl," Asia said as the two of them hugged each other.

The two of them started talking like Markus and I weren't even there. We just stood back, watching the expanding crowd while we talked about getting together for our business plans tomorrow.

"Jay, tomorrow night we should meet down at the Poetry Club downtown. You do have the rest of the weekend off from work, right?" Markus said.

With a sigh, I said, "Yes. I'm happy to get away from that sports bar for a whole weekend. The fact that the weekends are the busiest days there, I barely get weekends off."

"I know exactly what you mean about that. I've been working on a poem that I'm going to share with everyone at the Poetry Club tomorrow night. I go on at eight p.m."

"That's deep. I know you serious about your poetry and empowering black people. I will be there eight o'clock sharp."

"I invited Fred, but I doubt he will make it. He's probably somewhere now, dry humping every female in here with a phat ass."

After a light laugh at his comment, our conversation was interrupted by our ladies. They were ready to hit the dance floor. Kendrick Lamar's "Poetic Justice" was bumping out the speakers in a way that would persuade a preacher's wife to move to the music. Apparently, this song was the one that got our ladies ready to grind their Duncan Hines up against us until we were indeed ready to glaze their cakes. I found myself getting lost in my baby's fragrance again. Her scent was so mesmerizing that I pulled her near me. With her perky all-natural breast up against me, we just looked into each other with sex in our eyes. Without missing a beat, we grind to the beat of the music while my hands cupped her ass. In that moment I felt like freaking her right on the dance floor. In that very moment, the bat between in my pants was ready to hit a homerun, making sure I touched every base. Tonight, getting to third base wasn't good enough.

With my hardness increasing in my pants, I turned my baby around. I raised her right hand toward the sky as the DJ switched the song to Beenie Man's "Girls Dem Suga" which was one of my favorite reggae songs. This turned us up on the dance floor even more. She dropped down low then brought it back up while she danced to the music seductively. Moving to the wave of her hips, I sucked her earlobe as she continued to dance. I normally don't act like this in public, so I wasn't sure if it was the alcohol that was causing me to do exactly what I felt like doing.

Between me sucking on her earlobe, I said, "Follow me to the restroom."

With a questionable look, she said, "Why?"

"Woman, I got to piss, that's why, and I don't want your sexy self out here on the dance floor with these thirsty dogs."

"Okay, boo. They can look, but they know better than to touch. I will just wait for you near the restroom."

As my baby led the way to the restroom, we both walked our way through a jam-packed dance floor before we reached the restrooms. I walked closely behind her like my pelvic area was attached to her ass like conjoined twins. No one was going to have a chance to spit their best game to my girl tonight, or they would get a black eye. I tasted the wetness of my girl's lips before going into the men's restroom.

To my surprise, there was no one inside, which I thought was unusual, considering that niggas have been drinking and partying most of the night. After relieving some of the alcohol I consumed that night, I thought about doing something spontaneous. I had a certain urge to do what made me happy right then in that moment. Once again, the alcohol must be taking control of my body, because I didn't normally act spontaneously. My thoughts were usually premeditated.

Without another thought, I opened the restroom door and pulled Destiny by the arm to turn her around. Her face shone with so much elegance that I got lost admiring her beauty. Looking into her eyes was like looking into the eyes of heaven's angel. Softly kissing her lips while my hands raced up and down her spine, I felt my manhood throbbing to feel the moisture of her walls wrapped around it. Our tongues continued to wrestle each other as I tugged her into the men's restroom. She unzipped my shorts and started massaging the most sensitive muscle on my body with her hand. Without warning, she leaned her weight against me before giving me a big push. I stumbled into one of the bathroom stalls, watching her as she made her way toward me with a sense of urgency in her walk. Her body language said it all. She wanted this dick, and she wanted it right now. I was about to give her what she wanted in the best way.

I locked the door to the restroom stall while kissing her aggressively. One hand was now creasing her tits, and my other hand rose up her skirt to feel her warmth. Just like I thought, she didn't have any panties on. She pulled down my shorts as I lifted her up in the air. Her legs were around my waist, giving me an open invitation to go deep inside her sweet walls of bliss. With the fire and desire to feel myself deep inside of my girl, I rushed inside with long steady strokes. Her moans and wetness intensified as my strokes increased in speed.

Words weren't said, except for a bunch of gibberish that I interpreted as "This pussy is mine." I knew she was almost at her climax. Every time I hit that spot, her legs would start to shake while her eyes rolled in the back of her head like they were now. In that second, I started to feel my body getting tense, and I exploded inside her, releasing all my frustrations from having that damn conversation with my father.

As we both came back down to reality, we realized that there were other people inside the restroom with us now. We both laughed about it as we fixed our clothes.

"I wonder how long they'd been out there," Density said.

"I don't know, but I'm sure they got an earful," I said.

"Wait before you open the door. I need to wipe myself clean. You left a load in me. Good thing I'm on the birth control shots."

Even if she wasn't on the shots, I would probably still nut in her. I didn't think having a kid was a bad idea. I would finally prove to myself that I knew what it takes to be a father and show Samuel's ass that I was not anything like him.

"I wouldn't mind if you had my child," I whispered with a grin in hopes of disguising the seriousness in my voice.

"A baby isn't coming out of me without a ring on my finger," she replied, matching my tone with her own disguised sarcasm.

MORNING AFTER

My friends and I partied hard until the party was over at two in the morning. Overall, my family gathering and my girl's graduation party was a success. I had a blast. Throughout the day and night, I took photos with evidence that this day was something to remember. My best pictures from both parties were posted on my Facebook account for all my friends to see. Standing next to Destiny at the front door, thanking everyone for coming to her party, I was suddenly overcome with an overwhelming feeling of exhaustion. It was as if exhaustion wrapped me up like a mother wraps a blanket around her newborn. In this case, I didn't feel the love, warmth, and comfort as I would think a newborn would.

My skin was feelin' for a warm shower while my body was in need to feel the comfort of a soft bed and pillow immediately. It's a good idea that Destiny booked a room for us to sleep in at the Renaissance Hotel, which was walking distance from the club she rented. We both were too lazy to walk to the hotel, so I decided to drive us there.

In minutes after we walked into the room, we were both in the shower, washing each other's back, before crashing into each other's arms on the bed.

Several hours had passed, when I noticed the lingering smell of BBQ food was filling up the room. The aroma woke me up out of my sleep. Suddenly I had a flashback to the good food at my uncle's house. Now I was up, ready for some more. I reached for Destiny to pull her near me, only to discover I was alone in the bed now. Opening one eye at a time, my eyes witnessed what my arms discovered. Destiny was gone. A bit upset that she left before I could wake up, I reached for my phone to find out what's the time.

It's 9:30 a.m., so what's she doing up so early? Placing my phone down beside me, I noticed a note on her side of the bed, folded in half, facing down with my name written across it. I automatically knew that Destiny must have left the note for me explaining why she left so early. I quickly opened the note, curious to read why she left so suddenly in the morning:

> *Good morning, babe. I left early this morning around eight a.m. to go clean the club that I rented for my party. If I clean it up, they will reimburse me some of the money that I paid to rent the building. You know me. I'm going take that money to put towards having my own photo studio. Don't worry about helping because some of my closest friends are going help me clean. I left your plate of food in the microwave. Love you...Destiny!*

Reading the note made my prior feelings forgotten. I was feeling refreshed and ready to dive in this food that's in the microwave. After rinsing my mouth with some mouthwash that the hotel provided for their guests, I walked over to the microwave. I opened the microwave door, only to discover that Destiny ate half of my food.

"Damn that girl for eating half of my food," I said out loud as I picked up the plate of food out the microwave. Before I could start eating, I heard my cell vibrating. After a quick look at my cell, I noticed that it's my mama calling me. With my food in my hand, I walked over to the phone to answer it.

"Hello."

"Hello, son. Good morning. How are you?"

"Good morning. I'm fine, just eating some food from yesterday's BBQ."

"I know, because I can hear you chewing the food in your mouth. I told you don't chew with your mouth full, but in this case, I guess I will let you pass."

I could hear the sarcasm in her voice. My mama always knew how to make me smile when she wanted to. However, through her sense of humor, she was able to channel her serious mind.

"I'm over here getting ready for church. I wish you were here to go with me this morning."

Her statement marinated in my mind for a second. Now I knew the real reason why she called. She wanted me to start going to church with her. I could hear the gospel music playing in the background, indicating that she was praising God as she prepare for Sunday morning service.

"You know I'm nowhere near you, Mama. I'm all the way in Atlanta. Even if I were to decide to go to your church, I would have to make that decision at least a day in advance."

"Well, how about you make that decision a week in advance and come with me next week?" she said, barely giving me a chance to finish what I was saying.

"We been over this before, Mom. I feel as if I don't have to go to church every Sunday to have a relationship with God. There's people who are church leaders who doesn't even practice what they preach daily. And you know what, every Sunday they're at church while leaving the truth of who they really are lying in the dark."

"Don't allow one or a few sheep that went astray to cause you not to go and serve the Lord. I'm not judging you at all, son, but I do want you to join me at church sometimes. If you do have a relationship with God, I pray that he will show you that you must forgive your father."

At the minute I heard the word *father*, I stopped eating my food. I had to clench my teeth to stop myself from cussing while my mom was on the phone. My mom mentioning him made me experience serendipitous emotions that I'm not sure she understands. If she did, perhaps she wouldn't speak of him. Samuel Rodgers was the last person I wanted to think about right now, especially this early in the morning.

"Honestly, I'm not sure if I can forgive him right now. I don't want to think much about him at all. I have to get dressed and go to my dorm, so I will call you back later tonight before I meet Markus at the Poetry Club."

"I thought you were already at your dorm. And speaking of your dorm…now that you done with college, where you going to stay?"

"Markus and I discussing becoming roommates, so we're going to discuss that tonight. We want to be out of our dorm by next month."

"Okay, son, take care. I love you."

"I love you too…bye."

Hanging up the phone with my mom had me thinking that she will never let this forgiveness speech go. It's as if she forgot about how Samuel was never there. He would only come around whenever he wanted to. His attitude would change like the seasons. One minute he's around keeping everyone around him warm with his charm and smile. The next minute he leaves everyone cold and confused by his lack of consideration for other people's feelings. He's very undependable.

Physically he never hit my mom and me. Mentally, my faith in him becoming the father I hoped him to be has taken a beatin' over the years. If forgiving him was difficult for me, I just couldn't comprehend why it's so easy for my mom. I knew she knew that Samuel has committed adultery. I knew damn well a man is not going leave his woman at home for months at a time and not have other pussy somewhere else.

Maybe the only way I can learn to forgive was if I did start going to church. My mom was right. A few church leaders who have dabbled in the world of sin again don't mean I can't visit the house of the Lord to show thanks.

BUSINESS PLAN

On the way back from the hotel to my dorm, I could only think about enjoying my last day of relaxation before going back to work tomorrow evening. Working almost every weekend and going to class during the weekdays had been more than stressful. Not to mention the drive from one end of Atlanta to another can be hell due to traffic. Fortunately, I was finally able to get some free time to live a little. No more homework or midterms while balancing working as a waiter at TGI Friday's.

A nice drive on the highway seemed to be exactly what I needed because now that I made it to my dorm, I was feeling calm again. I just wanted to get in my dorm, take a shower, brush my teeth, put my things away, and watch TV. My bed was neatly made up like I left it. That was no surprise. However, I did notice mail lying on my bed, which indicates that my roommate must have received my mail by chance. His name was also Jordan, so sometimes our mail got mixed up.

"Hmmm! Should I open my mail now, or wait until I get out the shower?" I said out loud.

After contemplating shortly about whether I want to open my mail now or later, I decided to open it now. For all I know, it could be some more gift cards from friends and family. I love receiving gifts. The longer I stood there looking at the neatly wrapped envelopes on my bed, the more my curiosity to find out what was inside each envelope increased. Destroying the cover off each prized possession that lay beneath, I indeed felt like a kid again during Christmas. Smiling back at me, exposing their value, were gift cards and money. All these gifts had me feeling spoiled as hell right now. I had to make sure I personally let everyone know how grateful I was to receive gifts from all of them.

Now there was only one envelope left to tear open. *Samuel Rodgers* was written on the front of the envelope. Seeing his name almost made me rip the mail in half before opening it. Realizing he sent me something through the mail made me feel that he was just being devious. I know he said he sent me something in the mail, but you can never take his word seriously. Now I know that he was more than serious.

Slowly opening the mail in disbelief that I wasn't ripping to shreds anything that comes from Samuel, I became somewhat anxious to see what's inside. What can Samuel possibly give to me after he practically never stayed in my life full time? The opening of the mail left me in disbelief again. The item that I was pulling out the envelope left me stunned. In my hands lay a photo of Samuel holding me when I was a newborn. This photo had me in complete amazement. I never thought he cared about me enough to be around when I was born. My mom would tell me he was there, but I didn't believe it because he'd never been stable in my life. I just couldn't believe he was ever around to see me born since he never was around to see me grow into a man. Attached to the photo was a note.

> *Jordan,*
>
> *I want to start off by saying that I'm truly sorry that I wasn't there for you like a father should. I know you probably wondering why I sent you a photo of me holding you in the hospital. The answer is, I want you to know that although I made a mistake about not being a stable father figure in your life...I still was proud to see my first and only son. That day I held you in my arms for the first time was something that I will remember for the rest of my life. Like a punk I ran from responsibility because I was afraid I couldn't handle taking care of you and your mom. I'm sorry, and I know I can't make up for the time that was lost. I just want to spend the time we both have left to be there for you now. I love you...*

Could it be true that he's contrite? He sounded almost convincing. Maybe he was ready to attempt to rewrite all his wrongs by showing consistency. Just maybe I was ready to listen to what he had to say, especially if his action speaks louder than his words. Until then, I was going to enjoy spending this $200 prepaid card he sent me.

Now it was time for me to take that long, warm shower that I've been craving for. Quickly getting undressed as I gathered my rug and towel, I was more than ready to feel the water to cover my body. One second in the shower, I let out a sigh of relief. It's amazing the way water can cleanse a person in more ways than one. I felt like the steady rush of the warm water coming from the shower head was purifying my mind, body, and soul. This was my baptism in the Jordan River.

Waking up from a much-needed nap, I felt totally rejuvenated. I was ready for a nice evening at the Poetry Club. Those speaking poets at the club touched on some deep shit that made love to listeners' self-conscious thoughts. Each word penetrated the ear by the second while entering deep into your mind. And if listeners open themselves enough to the words, the message will enter deep inside their soul.

It's now seven o'clock. It would probably take me thirty minutes to get to the Poetry Club. I suppose, if I didn't already know what I wanted to wear tonight, I would be late. I hate being late on anything, so I quickly put on an orange Polo and beige shorts with some brown Polo shoes. After putting on some cologne, I checked the time once again to notice it's now 7:20. I still had time to update my Facebook page.

> *Come meet me at the Poetry Club tonight & allow the words of Markus, one the most talented poets I know, stimulate your mind. He will keep you coming back for more...trust me!*

I was sure that some of my Facebook friends that live in Atlanta will be in the building tonight. I knew for sure Markus will love that I tagged him in my Facebook message encouraging people to come see him perform. It was my way of showing some extra support besides showing up to the event.

Now 7:25, I was finally in my car, driving to the event. Thirty-five minutes was more than enough time to get there. *Maybe I should call my mom back while driving downtown, but then again maybe not.* I was not sure if I was in the mood to hear another lecture about church attendance or Samuel. Listening to music while driving was always therapeutic to me, so I just wanted to stay in the moment for a while longer. The deep wisdom of the poets at the club will only take my mind to another mellow place in time. Nearly two minutes away from the Poetry Club, I received a new text message. *Shit, I wonder who this is.* Quickly finding a parking spot, I grabbed my phone. I hit the power button to see who just texted me. Not only did I notice Markus texted me to tell me he's going on stage in three minutes, I also saw that it's now 7:57.

Damn. I better hurry up and get in this club. Fortunately, Markus put me on the VIP list so I didn't have to wait in line. I walked into a club that was small but seemed perfect for an intimate moment to share with someone you love or care about. The music was silky smooth that could place the most hostile person in tranquil mood.

The lights were low throughout the crowded club. Everyone seemed to be deeply engaged into what each poet had to say from the moment he or she walked on stage. It was something reminiscent of the poetry club in the movie *Love Jones*, except this spot had a small dance floor. I made it to the VIP section that's set up nearest the stage. Just as Markus was about to go on stage, I smiled because I made it on time.

Markus walked up to the side of the stage as his name was being introduced. Markus liked to dress up in character of whatever topic he was channeling for his poetry, so I wasn't shocked by his wardrobe. This nigga was wearing all-black leather jacket, black jeans, black boots, and a black hat. The outfit was something reminiscent of the Black Panther movement. He opened his mouth and began to speak words of knowledge:

> Throughout the early nineteenth century, people viewed things in color
> There was a black and white stigma that separated people of different color
> From the words of my mother, I will survive the storm
> The rain may fall, but my prayers will keep me from harm

> God gave Martin Luther King a dream so the people must follow
> People across the nation had to rise up, stand up against all barriers
> Stand tall, stand strong, stand with resilience
> Together we will fight the fight, together we will walk the walk, and together we will talk the talk
> Raise your fist in the air and remember the struggle…
> Throughout the twenty-first century people still view things in color
> No longer is it a black-and-white thing; instead it's a red-and-blue thing
> Gangs have corrupted the youth, thinking every argument has to end in a bang
> We went through the storm to get our freedom; now we're killing each other, taking our freedom
> The nation just can't seem to get past color barriers
> Aren't we all created equal? So let's respect one another
> Raise your fist in the air as we continue to fight through the struggle…

Everyone including me raised our fists in the air. We were touched by the poem. We all clapped in unison, showing credit to my nigga for writing such a powerful message.

Markus walked off stage to join me at the VIP table. We chest-bumped each other like mad animals in the jungle before sitting down. I couldn't imagine what others were thinking. They probably were looking at us with a bizarre look.

"Let's chill out and take a sit before everyone thinks we're crazy," I said.

Within an instant, Markus's body language changed as if an alarm went off inside him before we both sat down.

"Jay, you need to stop thinking about what others may think of you. Bruh, do whatever makes you feel happy. Do you think I was thinking about what someone else had to think of me when I didn't have sex with Quinesha years ago?" Markus said.

"No, Dad…calm down," I said, trying to lighten the mood.

I didn't understand it, but Markus sometimes took everything too seriously. Although I was serious about chilling out before people started looking at me crazy, I still didn't want him to concentrate on my self-conscious thoughts.

"I am calm. I just want you to start doing whatever it is that makes you happy. No one else can live your life for you…remember that."

"Okay, I will remember that. When we moving into our new apartment?" I said, changing the subject.

"Next month, in July…between the both of us, we have enough money saved to move in. We can move in the first week of July."

Suddenly Markus's mood changed again. This time he was smiling uncontrollably as he continued to talk. "It's the one we both wanted. The water bill is included in the monthly rent, so we can go half on the rent and light bill. Is that a bet?"

"Hell yeah! Markus, that's a bet!" I said without controlling my excitement.

I couldn't help but think how much I didn't want to move back in with my mom. I'd rather be independent, doing my own thing, instead of living under her roof again. *I'm far from a li'l boy. I'm a man now.*

"I know you didn't want to move back in with Mrs. Cheryl. I love my parents, but I don't want to move back in with them neither."

"You must read my mind, because I definitely don't want to move back with my mom. Who would want to move back to that small town our parents live in anyway?"

I watched Markus nod his head in agreement as he started to speak.

"Social Circle, Georgia, is a small town with zero opportunity for us to live out our dreams. There's no opportunity to grow and for us to accomplish what we're trying to build in a town that only have one red light."

We both laughed hysterically, because as odd as it sounded, what we said about Social Circle was true. That town was as country as it could get. There was no major attraction to the town, which equaled no growth, in my opinion. Every business that started there always failed. Our ultimate goal was to start a business that will grow, not shut down after a few months or years.

"I was thinking about the location we should place our first sports bar. Do you think we should buy a building outside of Atlanta?"

"That's a good question, Jay. I think we should take out a loan to buy a building outside the city, because I'm sure that will be cheaper than in the heart of Atlanta. I also think that it would be best to look for buildings that used to be a restaurant or bar that closed down. If we can find a decent building in a great location, money or time constraints won't be a problem."

"I totally understand. Buildings that used to be a restaurant would have at least a kitchen that we will need to prepare food for our customers. Plus it would most likely be spacious enough, so we can remodel the place to build a bar."

"If we find a building that was once a bar, it would be even better, because there's a possibility that we would have to do less repairing. We can then focus on décor of the bar more so than damn near tearing it down to rebuild it."

"I concur. Also I think we should target banks that will give us the best deals on loans once we narrow the buildings down. Once we get our business off the ground, then we discuss expanding."

"Unless we hit the lottery like the owner of this club…then we could start our own chain of sports bar," Markus said sarcastically.

This has turned out to be a productive night. Not only was I able to support my brother from another mother on a night he was given a spoken word, we were also able to talk about business. I felt like the DNA of our business plan was being structured right before our eyes. Once we find a bank to finance our business plan, the next step was to find the best building that's in the perfect location.

Looking at the time on my cell showed the time staring back at me along with a few Facebook notifications. Nearly two hours had gone by since I arrived at the Poetry Club. It's true what people say—time flies by when you're having fun. I was having such a great time listening to the poetic words of all the poets I completely lost track of time. Markus and I both lost track of time. We both promised our women that we would spend time with them tonight. I was surprised that neither one of our women blew up our phone while we were there. The fact that they didn't call only meant one thing: they must be together. Markus and I decided that we would have one more drink while listening to another spoken word from whomever steps up the stage.

As smooth jazz music faded in the background, I could hear more unknown conversations around me. The light on the stage appeared to shine brighter, signifying that someone must be coming to the stage. The anticipation crept into my blood stream, pumping its venom throughout my beating heart. My ears were ready to quench its thirst with the words of another potent message from a poet. I imagined this was how Jesus's twelve disciples felt every time he was about to speak.

The music was lowered as a tall light-skinned man with dreads beyond shoulder length walked on the stage with an engaging stage presence. This guy demanded attention based on his height and confidence alone. I was sure the ladies in the building tonight became moist between their legs once he walked on the stage. I mean, black women say that light-skinned men have gone out of style, but every time one of them sees a picture of Michael Ealy, their kitty cat drools. I was sure the women in the club were drooling now while their eyes were locked on the stage.

The words of this intellectual dude spoke to me in high volumes. He stood tall on the stage, speaking clear free of shame or nervousness. Not once did I sense a hint of shyness. This gave me the impression that this guy had spoken words in front of an audience many times before. His topic was about equality and the lack of it in today's world. I couldn't argue with the points he brought up, but it seemed like his words were subliminal. If I was not mistaken, he's suggesting that people need to stop discriminating against gays and lesbians.

> *Living in today's society, there's a new meaning to R. Kelly's "down low." Living in today's society, women can do some things in the light what others have to do in the dark.*

Those specific lines of his spoken word stood out to me. I was not sure if it's because of the passionate tone he carried in his voice or my curiosity to find out the depth of his message. Sounded like to me that he's a liberal man. If so, would that make him suspect to being gay? *Naw…I would know a gay man when I see it. I doubt he's gay.* I was sure he had a deeper meaning behind his words than I know.

HOME SWEET HOME

I was still thinking about the words of the last poet as I drove over to Destiny's apartment. She lived in midtown, so I knew it wouldn't take me long to get to her. At the moment, my mind wasn't quite driven on seeing her right now. I wouldn't tell her that. She wouldn't understand. Every time I leave the Poetry Club, there's always a poem that left me in deep thought. That's the reason why I loved going to the Poetry Club.

The equality poem by the young poet had me thinking about what if we lived in a world that everyone seriously has equal opportunities. If things really are equal, then people wouldn't live secret lives. The things that are said or done behind closed doors would be done when the doors are wide-open. The world has come a long way when it comes to equality among ethnic backgrounds. However, I couldn't help but think we have a long way to go. Even I was not comfortable with some things, such as homosexuality. I just didn't understand how someone could get sexual satisfaction from the same sex. Now the government was allowing certain states to marry the same sex. Perhaps my closed mind was not pressing equality but yet suppressing it with my scrutinizing thoughts.

Pulling into a parking space in my girlfriend's apartment complex, I remained in deep thought. It's like my mind was going at a speed of a thousand miles per hour. My thoughts were dictating the expressions that I have on my face, so I knew that when I stepped in Destiny's apartment, she was going to ask me that infamous question: *what's wrong with you?* She's notorious for asking questions I didn't want to answer, especially when she could tell something's wrong. Tonight I was not sure if I was ready to answer that question, but it's a part of the inevitable.

I placed the key in the door handle and walked right into Destiny's colorful world. The décor of her apartment was beyond dull. Destiny was into fashion and colors, so her place indicated that she was not afraid of color by any means. The living room was basically different shades of red, yellow, with a hint of black. *GQ* and *Vogue* magazines, as well as other fashion magazines, neatly covered the middle of her coffee table. As she looked through a magazine, I could tell she was enjoying her study of what's the latest fashion trend. Without saying anything, I sat down beside her.

With her eyes still infatuated by the perfectly edited photos in the fashion magazine, she still somehow managed to read my body language.

"What's wrong with you," Destiny said.

With teeth clenched tightly, I took a moment to think about whether I wanted to discuss everything on my mind with her. Maybe it wouldn't be a bad idea to discuss the equality poem. I was kind of interested to know what would be her perspective on the subject.

"I'm just thinking about this equality poem that I heard at the Poetry Club. It has me thinking about how different the world would be if everyone could live without shame of what they like," I said.

She placed the magazine down with one eyebrow raised. Now her body language was insinuating that I have her full attention.

"Elaborate."

"You know how people say what's done in the dark will come to the light. Well, if we all treat each other equally, there won't be a need to do things in the dark that someone will feel ashamed to do in the light."

"Right…I also think that the only way that everyone is treated equally is if we're perfect. Being perfect would eliminate the chances of imperfections, which would mean no one would be sinfully judged. The truth is, no one's perfect, so there's always going be someone who's not going to like someone because of the way they look, something they did or said. Fashion models and celebrities get tough criticism every single day. That's why my passion is to work behind the scenes as a photographer. I just can't deal with the judgmental comments all the time," she said.

I wasn't stunned at all in hearing my baby say this, although she's a very strong person. I believed even the strongest people have a breaking point. You have to know what it feels like to be weak or broken to learn what it takes to be strong. There's no such thing as being too strong, because new challenges are bound to come.

"You so right, babe. I couldn't deal with the stress of being in the spotlight, living the lavish life every single day either," I said as I placed her legs across my lap. "Markus and I found a new place to call home sweet home, by the way."

She looked at me while I read the joy in her eyes matching the smile on her face.

"Jordan! I'm so proud for the both of you. When y'all moving in?"

"Markus and I are moving next month off Briarcliff Road. We also talked about our business plans. Opposed to searching for a building downtown, we going to start out finding a spot outside of downtown—the prices will be more reasonable."

"Let me know if there's anything I can do to help. Maybe I can take some random photos of people playing sports and use it to decorate the sports bar."

I shook my head in disagreement.

"I rather have photos of the world's most famous sport figures stamped on the walls of Markus's and my establishment than to have some dusty-ass wannabe Michael Jordan on the walls of my sports bar."

She kicked me playfully in the stomach while she covered her mouth, trying to hide her laughter.

"That was kind of mean of you to say."

"Umm hmm…whatever you say."

After the laughter died down, Destiny became more serious. Her facial expression read that she had something to tell me that she didn't know how.

"What's wrong?" I said as I massaged her feet and looked deep into her eyes.

With a sigh of hesitation, she said, "You know I'm into graphic design and photography. My dream is to own a photo studio as well as becoming a major photographer."

"Yes, we discussed this before, so why you looking so distraught?"

"I guess it's because I, umm…thinking about moving back to my home city of Detroit now that college is over. I would rather build my brand of photo studios right in my home city before branching out to other major cities."

A part of me wanted to tell her hell no, she can't go…that she can start her career right here in Atlanta first. I mean, this is a better market than Detroit. Shit! Detroit ain't known for fashion, modeling, or photography anyway. Destiny should know that Atlanta is a better market to start a photo studio than Detroit. I would understand if she was launching her career in New York City or LA instead of trying to live out her dream in a city of lost hope. Although I never visited Detroit, I knew that the city went down after automobile companies suffered from the economy setback. Across the United States, every city and small town was affected by the economy, but it just seemed like the city of Detroit sunk the most.

Here I was, thinking that she would start her career in Atlanta up until now. I guess it's what they call a rude awaking. I wanted to tell her that I didn't understand why she wanted to go back to what seemed to be a piss-poor city that hardly had shit going on for itself, but instead, I spoke the opposite.

"I totally understand. We both have dreams that we want to start in our home state before branching out across other parts of the States. I support you. What about us?"

"I've given everything some serious thought. I absolutely know the odds we will face shifting from a short-distance relationship to a long-distance relationship. It's something I sincerely feel we can not only conquer but also endure any obstacles that may stand in the way."

As I sat there watching my girl wipe away a tear from her eye, I wanted to beg her to stay like a drunken Keith Sweat fan. I wanted to sing at the top of my lungs every whiney Keith Sweat song in hope that it would convince her to stay. Although I wanted to tell her I loved her and I would miss her if she goes, my pride kept a grip on my tongue. The humiliation of looking soft glued my mouth shut.

Less than thirty days we both would be home sweet home. The only difference was, I would be claiming a new place to call home in the state I was born and raised. On the other hand, she would be going back to a place that she'd known as home for years. We both would start a new chapter in our lives miles apart. I hoped to one day have enough courage to tell her how I really felt about her.

LONG DISTANCE

Five months had passed by since the last time I'd seen my Destiny. Only I knew that since my Destiny was gone, I'd been living without a purpose. The days throughout the summer when I was hot, she wasn't there to cool me down. On the cold nights in December, she's not there to keep me warm. Instead I lay in my bed alone, snuggled underneath my covers, contemplating how much more of this loneliness I could take. We talked on the phone daily about life, goals, and accomplishments. Sometimes we even used Skype, but nothing was like having her near me.

I just wanted to feel another body next to mine, with long hair, perky breast with ripe nipples, and a nice ass. If I hit up a freak on Facebook that went to Clark Atlanta with me, would that be such a bad idea? A part of me didn't think so, because I would love to feel a warm, wet mouth swallowing my manhood at this very moment. Five months in this long-distance relationship I'd been faithful, but the temptation had been hard to resist. The thought of being in this predicament had made me at times want to resent Destiny. The only thing that won't allow me to resent her was the fact that I did love her.

My raw emotions about this long-distance situation remained hidden from strangers easily. The ones who really know me knew I was bruised inside. I suppose that's why Markus kept telling me that I should release my inner thoughts through poems. I heard him. I actually thought writing poems expressing how I truly felt will be therapeutic, but I wouldn't know where to start. My thoughts were going through my head faster than a speeding bullet.

Day to day I battled with my mind, trying to suppress these emotions I kept balled up inside. Slightly losing concentration of getting closer to my dreams of being a successful businessman, I felt as if I was letting my business partner down. Markus had been pulling most of the weight trying to get our business plans off the ground. The banks were being cautious about who they're allowing to borrow money. I believed it's because the economy and all the foreclosures on homes didn't help them trust giving money out to loaners. We've also been having a hard time finding the perfect building to buy for our business ventures.

With everything going on in my personal and business life, I've become stressed. I needed to release some of this pressure that's lying heavily on my chest.

"Damn! What the!" I yelled out loud as I felt something vibrating under the top part of my back.

It was my cell phone. I left it on vibrate since last night. I remember falling asleep with it beside me, but somehow it must have gotten under me. I left it on vibrate hoping that it wouldn't distract me from my thoughts, but it still found a way to do so. Depending on whose number showed up on the ID, I would answer.

Looking at my phone, the name Destiny popped up with her picture. Without hesitation, I answered the phone. Just the thought that I was about to hear her voice had ounces of blood rushing from my head to the lower part of my body. Now my other guy was up and ready to come out to play.

"Hello," I said.

"Hello, babe. I was just thinking about you," Destiny said in a seductive tone.

"At four a.m. in the morning…so tell me what got you thinking about me?"

At this point, I knew where this conversation was going, so I pulled my boxers down. Jacking off was something that I expected every teenage boy to do at some point, even if they're too embarrassed to admit it. Honestly, I was starting to fall back in love with doing it because somehow it's helping me remain faithful to my relationship with Destiny. I just was not sure how long this will be enough, but it will have to be good enough for now.

Although I wanted to see her…touch her, instead I just listened to her mesmerizing voice as I remembered visions of her naked body lying on my bed. As my babe rested her weight on her elbows with her back and legs arched, face looking up toward the ceiling, I continued to kiss her neck. While her eyes closed, I spread her legs apart, leading my way to the inside of her thighs. With two fingers, I massaged her clit gently, touched every angle of her lips below. With each touch, I made her moan. With every moan, it made me want to beat it with the rigidness that was between my legs. I imagined that it was soaking wet inside her deepest walls based on the moisture that was on my fingertips. Before I could get into position, her legs began to tremble, indicating that she's about to reach her first climax. Being the freak that I was, I slid my beef cake inside so I could feel the wetness and warmth of her cum as I stroked her deep.

"I'm about to cum, baaabbbeee!" Destiny said, slightly snapping me back into reality.

For a minute I was in such a trance reminiscing about one of our last sexual encounters I forgot that it was only a memory, not reality. The night before she moved back to Detroit, we had some of the best lovemaking. I was not sure if it was because we both knew it would be the last time for a while, but I just knew that it was very intense. Now all I can do was reminisce about it while having phone sex. I got to see her soon.

"I feel that nut, baby. Damn!" I said.

"I love you."

"I love you too."

As if Destiny was having another orgasm, she inhaled with extreme force. I could imagine her looking stunned at me with her mouth open, hand placed on her heart. She might not know it, but I was as stunned as she was that those three words came out my mouth. In the past I told her "You too" when she said she loved me; I never actually said the words *I love you*. After my graduation party with my family, I told myself I would express to her how much she meant to me, but I couldn't build up enough courage to do so. I guess it's something about the distance that somehow brought me closer to her emotionally.

The distance had placed its wrath down on me to the point I couldn't deny how I really felt about my Destiny.

"Did you just say what I think you said?" Destiny said with joy and disbelief.

"Yes. I said it. Don't act all surprised. You know that I care about you."

"I know, but hearing you say it makes this a special moment. I'm a strong believer in 'Actions speak louder than words,' but there's always a desire to hear the words along with the action."

"I agree with that. Well, I'm going to go take another shower since you had me make a mess all over myself. I will talk to you later on today."

"Okay…talk to you soon. I love you. Bye."

"I love you too. Bye."

As we hung up, I could hear the excitement in her voice that I finally said those three words. Those three words pack a mighty powerful punch. Once it hits you, it's going to leave you either in pain or in joy. It might even make you feel both pain and joy. Like I heard Al Green sing plenty of times before on my mom's records, *love will make you do wrong…love will make you do right*. I have a feeling that one day I will find out what that's all about.

TAKING A CHANCE

Now that I've confessed my love to Destiny, I wondered if I should move to Detroit, Michigan. It's evident that I'm lovesick without her. Admitting to myself that I love her and saying it out loud was a big step for me. Perhaps I was ready for a change. I mean, a change of scenery couldn't be that bad of an idea. We discussed the possibility of me moving to Detroit. Stepping out on faith, I believed that it's time that I move where my girl's at. Moving hundreds of miles away from Atlanta would place strain on Markus's and my business endeavors. As business partners, we're having a challenging time finding a building that meets our budget as well as what we desire in a building. I doubt he will be happy about conducting business back and forth from long distance. He always told me I have to start doing what makes me happy, so this time I thought I was going to finally take his advice.

My adrenaline rush was working overtime, forcing me to react differently than I was accustomed to. My elation for my decision may seem uncommon for others who know me, but to me, it's my revelation for a brand-new start. I was taking a chance in life. My fresh start would be surrounded by familiarity. The climate of the Midwest would be something that I will have to adjust to. Thank God I will have my Destiny to warm. She would be my familiarity in a foreign place. I could almost smell the fragrance of my girl's distinct scent running across my nostril, her scent blowing through the breeze as we walk through the park, holding hands like we can never be apart.

Instead of waiting, I was just going to shower my Destiny with the good news now before she goes to sleep. With my phone in my hand, I anxiously called my girl phone. After three rings, she answered with sleep evident in her voice.

"Hello," she said.

"I have good news," I said.

"What is it?"

"I've decided to move to Detroit."

"What...what about you coming to visit first before making that decision?"

I could feel her excited even though she was hundreds of miles away. We never lived together before, but I was ready for that step in our relationship. I hoped she was ready for it too.

"I didn't want to overthink it. I mean, I love you and you love me, so why not?"

"You're right, but it's just unorthodox of you to make a spontaneous decision on your own."

We both said good night to each other one more time before we hung up. Looking up at the ceiling as I lay on my bed, I wondered how I was going to break the news to my family and my business partner. *Maybe I should tell Markus in the morning. I could tell my family at the Christmas party this week. I can put in my two-week notice at my job this week also so they can find a replacement. Everything will work itself out.*

As the morning sun peeked through my blinds, I imagined it yelling to me, "Wake ya ass up!" One glance at my clock, now I noticed it's not morning, but it's early in the afternoon. I was sure Markus was up by now. Hopefully he's still at home so we could talk about the business and the effects my move will have on the business. I was sure he will understand why I decided to move. With work starting in a couple of hours as well as wanting to have this important talk with my roommate, I needed to get up right now. There's no time for procrastination.

A slow hop out the bed, I started to make my way to my bathroom. Every morning, brushing my teeth and washing my face were my first priority. After finishing my morning rituals, I made my way toward the kitchen. Markus was lying on the couch, watching Sports Center. He didn't look like he'd been anywhere today, wearing basketball shorts and wifebeater.

"You haven't been out today," I said.

"Naw. Not today. I have the day off, so I decided to chill," Markus said.

"I talked to Destiny early this morning. We discussed our future together. I finally admitted to her that I love her."

Instantly Markus stopped watching the TV. Markus's face spoke volumes, that he's in total disbelief. Although he knew how I felt about Destiny, I never told her or anyone that I loved her. Markus was one of the few people who knew how well I hide my true emotions in the dark. He always told me to speak my mind; fuck what others think of me.

"That's a huge step for you, bruh."

"A huge step indeed. I'm also considering moving to Detroit next month. I wanted to run across you because you're my business partner as well as my closest friend. I would love to have your blessings."

The TV has lost Markus's attention completely as he rose up from lying down to look me dead in my eye as he began to speak once again.

"I know you love Destiny. Have you thought this through?"

"Yes, I've been thinking about it. Destiny and I thought it would be best if I visit Detroit first before making a permanent decision about moving. Moving to the Midwest is somewhat a big commitment that we both need to be ready for. After craving to see her and be around her, I just decided what the hell. I might as well take a chance. I feel it's worth it."

"As long as you thought about what you walking into, then I definitely couldn't dispute the idea of you moving. Are y'all going to move in together?"

"We explored the possibility of me moving to Detroit. We both agreed that moving together is an option as well as a big-ass commitment. I'm not sure how well the experience of living together's going be…man, I never lived with anyone I was in relationship with before. We agreed that we going to move together."

"Right. What about our business?"

"I know that our business plans haven't shaped up the way we imagine. The fact I'm talking about moving don't help the situation at all. However, I do believe that we can still make it work. We can always do video conferences with one another. While I'm living in Detroit, I don't plan on stop hustling to get our business up and running. In fact, I think I'll become enthusiastic again about our dreams once I get closer to my girl."

"I totally agree, because how you been walking like you a grumpy old man has been aggravating sometimes. I wanted to slap the shit out you in hope that you would snap out of it."

We both laughed hysterically. My right-hand man was right. I was trying to hide my feelings, but he always saw right through all the bullshit I tried to use to cover up my sentiments. We've been friends for years.

"A'ight…a'ight…a'ight…enough of the clowning, you clown-ass nigga."

We gave each other dab, which was our own sign of reaching an agreement. I just hoped that breaking the news to my family goes this smooth. My mom probably will take it the hardest, because she never had to deal with me not being in driving distance from her. She just would have to understand that I was not a baby no more. It's time I made grown-man decisions. I couldn't live my life according to how others wanted me to forever, although most of my life I did. One day soon, I hoped to live my life the way I wanted to without wondering what someone else thinks about me.

CHRISTMAS PARTY

It's Christmas, the twenty-fifth of December, what many claim to be the jolliest day of the year. The weather outside was cold and slightly windy unlike the Midwest or up north. Down south we don't receive much snow. Wintertime in Georgia usually gives us black ice on the roads as opposed to snow on the roads. Whenever it did snow, you can bet everyone who's from Georgia is reluctant to drive. People who are from up north usually try to drive on the roads anyway because they feel like us Southern folks don't know how to drive.

As a kid I loved for it to snow. I knew if snow was on the roads, school would be canceled. Besides school being canceled, I would love to see a crazy person trying to drive in the snow. Usually every time they tried, they would get stuck. I thought it was pure comedy. My childhood memories of seldom getting snow were good times, but it can't snow today. The snow would interfere with my family Christmas party. Besides the fact I had big news to share with my family, this could be one of the last family gatherings I was a part of for a while. Once I moved to the Midwest, I was not sure when or how often I will be able to come back.

The party was over my Uncle Joe's house in East Point, Georgia, as usual. He had the biggest house out of everyone in the family, so it's fitting to have family celebration over his crib. My favorite uncle didn't seem to mind. Every time we have a party at his crib, we have so much fun. We didn't spend Thanksgiving together as a family, so this was the last time we'd all be together since my graduation celebration. Besides turning up with my family, I didn't know how I was going tell them about my expected move. I was not sure how everyone will take the news. I could only hope that everyone will be happy for me.

Arriving at my uncle's crib, I could tell that the party has started without me. There was a plethora of vehicles in the yard as well as by the side of the curb. My nerves were on edge about breaking the news about moving to another state. Usually driving while listening to Mary J. Blige composes me like a cigarette does to a nicotine fiend. However, today what usually my nicotine was not keeping me calm. Instead I was more anxious than ever to get it over with now that I was finally there. Before grabbing the presents and gifts cards, I noticed all the ladies in the living room.

Before I could ring the doorbell, Aunt Bev opened the door with a huge smile on her face. Her smile was so huge you would think she's looking at her celebrity crush. Wearing her black-and-pink pant outfit, she was certainly looking comfortable but yet dressed for the occasion. Aunt Bev loved her pink, so I didn't expect her to wear Christmas colors even on Christmas Day.

"Hello, Aunt Bev, you didn't give me a chance to ring the doorbell," I said.

"Suga', I saw you when you parked outside. Your mom and I, along with others, are sitting in the living room, watching holiday movies. The men are down in the game room watching basketball," she said.

I walked right in while Aunt Bev held the door open for me. I was sure she was eyeing the presents in my arms, hoping that one of them was hers. She didn't have to worry because one of them was hers indeed. Aunt Bev was like a second mother to me. I wouldn't feel right not buying her something for Christmas.

"Aunt Bev, I have a present for you. I know it's not Denzel Washington wrapped in a huge box, but this will have to do," I managed to say through a chuckle.

Aunt Bev's celebrity crush, as long as I can remember, has been Denzel Washington. She owned all his movies. I knew Uncle Joe got jealous sometimes. The expressions on his face when Aunt Bev talked about how fine she thought Denzel was, was written all over his face in bold ink.

"Suga', there's not a better present than Mr. Denzel Washington himself, but I will kindly take what you give me."

Aunt Bev let out a light laugh before giving me a huge hug, rocking me from side to side. As I was close to her so no one would notice, I whispered in her ear not to open her present around everyone. I had bought her some expensive perfume from Macy's. I didn't want everyone to see her gift then ask me why I didn't buy them something from Macy's.

I started a Christmas savings every year around January so I was able to buy gifts for my family. Unfortunately, not everyone in my family was able to get the most expensive gifts. I can only do so much when it comes to playing Santa Claus for a day. After giving out the envelopes to everyone, I made sure that I greeted everyone with love. I had bought majority of the women a twenty-dollar gift card from Bath & Body Works. How could you go wrong with giving a woman a gift card for a feminine store that sells perfume, scented lotions, soap, and candles? I love to put a smile on people's face, especially the ones I love. Speaking of the ones I love, I couldn't wait to give my gift to my mom as I watched her approach me with a generous smile.

"Merry Christmas, Mom…I love you. I have a present for you."

"Why, thank you. Regardless if you buy me material things or not, blessing me with your presence is more than enough for me," she said with her arms wrapped around me.

It's safe to say that I'm a mama's boy. She has been there for me as long as I can remember. There's no way to repay her for how supportive she's been in my life. She always wanted the best for me. I wanted the best for her because she deserved the best. With a smile bigger than Santa Claus's belly, I gave my mom her presents. Patiently waiting for her to open the envelope, I was boiling over with anticipation to see her reaction. Calmly my mom opened the first envelope to witness two tickets to the Gospel Music Fest.

"Lord have mercy! I was praying to the Lord about these tickets, son. I miss the Gospel Music Fest every year! Hallelujah! Thank you, Jay."

My eagerness for my mom to open her next gift was pouring out of me like smoke out of a volcano. I didn't know whether to jump, shout, or just be unruffled by the emotion I was feeling inside.

I said as calmly as I could, "Okay, Mom, don't get overly excited. You still have another envelope to open."

Instead of calmly opening the second envelope, she impatiently opened the next one. Standing in front of my mom, I could feel the excitement of finding out what her next surprise gift was going to be. It was like static electricity. I knew she would love this gift equally as the first one. It always was a pleasure to see my mom smile. Often in the past, I'd seen her broken and mentally drained from the relationship with Samuel. I never understood how a man could be so cold toward the mother of his child. That was more than enough reason why I tried to put a smile on my mother's face more than anything. As I watched how elated she was at this moment, I smiled.

"Oh! Jay, you shouldn't have…reservations to a spa. I don't know what to say."

"You don't have to say much, Mama. I just want to see you happy."

After my mama and I had our made-for-TV moment, I made my way to the game room with the fellows to watch some basketball. Halfway near the game room, I could hear my cousins and uncles were all the way turned up. If I didn't know better, I would've thought they were in there fighting. Anytime there were sports, food, and alcohol involved with more than five men in a room, that's the formula for a testosterone overflow.

Walking into the room, I saw what women would see as chaos while men would view as acting normal. A big-ass seventy-two-inch high-definition television was displaying the most crystal-clear picture that money can buy. I always love watching sports on my Uncle Joe's television. The atmosphere with the fellas was extremely different. This was what I was accustomed to when I was with my cousins and uncles during game time. Eating, drinking, laughing, and talking shit were what we do best when watching any sports. I just got to get me a beer out the small refrigerator so I can join in on the shit talking these niggas were doing. One thing I learned though is that no one can talk more shit than my Uncle Joe.

"What! Nigga, you can't tell me he didn't travel. Robert, now you know you my baby brother, but I swear you got the eyes of an old bat trying to find his way in the daylight," Uncle Joe said.

"Fuck you! Joe! I bet this old bat can still beat your ass in a game of basketball," Uncle Robert replied with a loud aggressive tone matching his brother's.

Everyone laughed in unison. Getting caught with the entertainment of the game as well as the humor of my Uncle Joe and Uncle Robert's debate, I almost overlooked how much weight Uncle Joe lost. Since the last time I saw him, he told me he's going to start eating healthy in an effort to lower his high blood pressure. I didn't know how dedicated to a new diet he would be.

Not knowing exactly what to give the fellas on Christmas was something I struggled with every year. Men are simple when it comes to gifts. They don't usually ask for much, so I usually just hand out gift cards to a restaurant where they can order a steak or gift cards to a sports bar. *I will just hand out their cards when the game goes to halftime.* The second quarter was coming to a close now. *Maybe it would be a good idea to tell the fellas about my plans to move to Detroit. It would be easier to tell them than the women of my family.*

I was sure all the women will be crying like it's a funeral. There's no need for tears. The only thing dying was my past, because next month, I was going start a new future in a new part of the United States. I truly couldn't wait.

The game went into halftime as Aunt Bev walked through the door almost simultaneously. She had an apprehensive look on her face like she had something to say. No one else seemed to notice her come in the room just like they didn't notice me. They were all so engaged in their shit talking to focus on anything around them. Aunt Bev seemed to notice how deeply involved they were with debates, so she stood in front of the TV and turned it off to gather everyone's attention. Instantly everyone looked at her with astonished look on their faces.

"Cheryl has an announcement to make. She wants everyone to be around when she reveals what her announcement is," Aunt Bev said.

"You better be glad it's halftime, woman. Coming in her with your nosy ass talking about a big announcement," Uncle Joe said to his wife in aggravated tone.

"Awww! Shut up, Joe, I checked on the television in the living room to see if halftime was about to start before coming down here. Your baby sister got something to say, so bring your ass to the living room."

I don't know about anyone else, but I was eager to hear what my mom has to say. The fact that she wanted to tell everyone at the same time made me even more curious. Once everyone made it into the living room, my mom stood at the center. She was officially the center of attention. The big grin on her face and what seemed to be a glow on her skin were enticing my curiosity even more. I've seen my mom overwhelmed with joy before. However, I don't recall her being overwhelmed with joy like that in a long time.

Respectfully, I made my way toward the front of everyone to make sure I hear the words that will come out my mama's mouth without misinterpretation. Right before she began to speak, she laughed like a li'l girl who was around her secret crush.

"I want to thank everyone for gathering around as I reveal something that's important in my life. Prior to today, it took everything in me to keep my secret this long. Enough of the small talk. I'm happy to invite everyone to a wedding on New Year's Eve."

The whole room got quiet with confusion because everyone knew that Mom was still married to Samuel. There's just no way she was deciding to renew her vows. She couldn't be serious about marrying this punk-ass husband of hers a second time. Releasing my clenched teeth, I spoke out with rage in my voice before I knew it.

"Are you insinuating that you're going to renew your vows with that punk-ass husband of yours?"

"Jordan Rodgers, I raised you to never disrespect adults in this manner, especially not me, so be careful what you say around me, boy. You might think you grown, but I will still get on the butt." Rolling her neck while pointing her finger my direction, she went on to say, "And for your information, yes, I am renewing my vows with your father."

"You know what, while we're revealing big announcements, I have one of my own. I'm moving to Detroit next month. Now that I'm hearing about a renewing of vows, I think it's time that I leave."

Without listening to another word, I gathered my belongings and headed to the front door. I refused to hear about a bullshit renewing of a marriage that should've been over a long time ago. How could she go back to someone who did nothing but neglect her when things wasn't convenient for him? To make matters worse, she's running back to him with open arms. Does she really think that I would accept it? I felt betrayed.

NEW BEGINNING

My first winter in Detroit was brutally cold. No matter how cold I thought the Motown city was, nothing compared to the cold I experienced last Christmas. Hearing the words "I am renewing my vows with your father" coming out of my mom's mouth sickened me. I was truly livid from what seemed to be the worst decision she could've made. Literally her decision seemed like a sharp knife stabbing me in my heart, causing it to bleed anger and frustrations.

I was so bothered by Mom's decision that night. Six months later, I was still tortured by her devastating announcement. Still being upset about the renewal of their marriage, not only did I not attend the wedding, I also didn't speak much to my mom at Markus's wedding. Samuel and Cheryl Rodgers had the audacity to show up all over each other like newlyweds. It was just damn right ridiculous how they were all over each other like horny drunken teenagers. He tried to hold a conversation with me, but I quickly walked away. I will admit, after his graduation gift, I did feel like our relationship could be repaired. Healing from a disappointing childhood, when Samuel should've been the father figure in my life, was something that will take time for me to get over. The part-time father figure remarrying my mom didn't help me get over the disappointment of him playing my father temporarily.

Here I am today, trying to prove to someone that was hardly around that I can be a better father than him. My birthday just passed a month ago in May. As opposed to enjoying my youthful life partying and drinking, living life carefree, I'm wondering why Destiny won't agree to have my baby. She must not understand that this is deeper than her having a career. She's always throwing up in my face that she wants to focus on her career, not raising a baby. Then she gets on the subject of marriage and how she wants to be married before having a baby. Fuck that shit she's talking. I always do what others want or what I think others want me to do. Instead of thinking about what anyone else wants, I'm going to think about what I want, for a change. I've placed myself in the backseat for too long as I watched others take control of the wheel. Now it's my time to drive this relationship and my life in the direction I want it to go. I'm finally taking over the wheel. The old way of decision making is out the window while a new beginning has flown in.

"Damn it! Jay! You always bring up having a son. I don't feel like hearing a goddamn lecture about having your baby today," Destiny says with furious hand gestures and facial expressions.

Not backing down, I say with bass in my voice, "Well, you going hear it today, so you might as well listen!"

"You need to be focusing more on living out your dreams of owning a sports bar instead of settling for working at one. We both are young adults with the potential to be successful with accomplishing our dreams. Bringing a child into the equation right now will be too much of a burden for the both of us. Just think rational."

"I am thinking rational. We can balance a career and raise a child. People do it all the time. My mother did it for years by raising me."

"Okay, Jordan, but guess what. You ain't your mother, and neither am I. When I'm ready to focus on starting a family, I will. I don't need the pressure from you or anyone to convince me otherwise. A true commitment with a diamond ring on this finger will have to come before having anyone's baby."

"You're right…you ain't my mother. I think we should leave her out of this before I say something you wouldn't want to hear."

With her hands clutch into tight fists at her sides, she says, "Something I wouldn't want to hear? What the fuck that supposed to mean, Jordan? Keep popping off at the mouth, I will show you how Detroit bitches get down."

With that statement, I let her have the last words before things got physical. We would argue, but I would always walk away before things got out of hand. Although there're moments when I want to slap her like some random hoe on the street, I never could do it. Instead of hitting her, I walk out our bedroom into the living room. Sometimes the bedroom we share feels like a box ring where we both hit each other below the belt with words. Deep down inside, I still have a lot of love for her even though some of that love is lost.

Prior to moving with her, I thought things would be better between us, but over the months, things somehow got worse. In the past, we never argued the way we do now. Now when we make love, I use that as an opportunity to be rough with her. Instead of her backing down, it seems to turn her on more. I used to be more gentle, touching and caressing her body like fine china. Now I find myself releasing my aggravations on her through pulling and smacking her ass multiply times from the back during sex.

Regardless of what's going on with us, I can't shake the feeling that my new beginning here in Detroit may turn out to be the beginning of the end of our relationship.

BUSINESS PROPOSITION

About thirty minutes went by since the confrontation with Destiny. Now I'm feeling calm. Although my feelings about having a child remains the same, I've collected my thoughts about the situation as I sit in the living room in a laid-back mood, feeling like tranquility came and wrapped me up in her arms. Relaxation has crept, causing me to drift off to my dream world. Everything seems to be perfect in my dream world. This place of imagination always seems to be perfect, filled with happy endings.

Living the lavish life in a luxury home with some of the finest cars anyone could lay eyes on, my Destiny by my side, with our kids next to the both of us as we get ready for a family day out on a warm sunny day—no worries or regrets. Not only will my sports bar be thriving, but Destiny's career would be blooming as well.

Drifting back into reality, I hear Destiny calling my name. *Damn! I wonder what she wants now.*

Looking up at her, I notice she's standing behind the sofa, towering over me. She doesn't speak with hostility, instead she speaks hastily. I don't know what's the matter now.

"Did you forget we're having company come over?"

Looking up at here with a bizarre face probably explains that I completely forgot about her inviting someone over for me to meet. All she told me was she has a client that works in the finance department for a major bank.

"My bad. I will admit I did forget your client was coming over. What he coming over for?"

"Like I told you before, you will have to find out when he gets here. He's at the door, so I'm going to go let him in. Go sit at the dining table. We will meet you there."

"A'ight, cool."

As I begin to walk out the living room, I stop in front of the long mirror hanging on the wall to straighten up my baby-blue shirt. For some reason, Destiny wanted us to dress up. I'm assuming this must be some sort of business meeting. She has on a high-waist skirt with a golden sleeveless top with her expensive Jimmy Choo shoes that her parents bought her last Christmas. Meanwhile, I complied with dressing in some khaki pants with some chocolate Tom Ford shoes she bought me for my birthday.

This agreement to meet here for a business meeting doesn't surprise me one bit. Destiny loves showing off her luxury apartment. Her parents are very wealthy, so her standards when it comes to her living condition have always been pertaining to the upper class. I tend to think that any apartment can be fixed up to look like you're living in luxury. That goes for any apartment that isn't in the hood. Destiny, along with her baby brother and older sister, doesn't know how good they got it made. My mom could never afford to spoil me with material things growing up or even now to this day. I had to be ambitious and work diligently to get everything I have. Destiny's brother and sister are spoiled rotten like they're the only child, when in reality, I'm the one who grew up as the only child. I'm definitely not an example of children growing up without siblings who are spoiled rotten.

Destiny's apartment is located near downtown Detroit. The exquisite apartment has a fireplace, two walk-in closets, two baths, and two bedrooms. She isn't doing bad for an aspiring photographer and business owner. It seems like she has clients booked for a photo shoot every hour. Every photo shoot she books gets her closer to starting her own photo studio. Then she can finally work for herself instead of the jealous boss she works for at the photo studio in the mall. Her boss is so jealous of her work and the clients she brings in. Women can be so catty.

Finally making to the dining table with its multicolored chairs, I sit down, waiting for Destiny and her guest to arrive at the dining table. The laughter and footsteps start to get closer to me. Whoever this person is must be someone she likes, because she seems to be having the conversation of her life.

As the two approach the dining table, I notice this guy is extremely tall. His dreads are pulled back, exposing his baby face with a well-groomed goatee, blue eyes reminiscent of the actor Michael Ealy. I've seen him somewhere before; I just can't remember where.

Rising up from my seat with my hand extended, I say, "Hey, man. I'm Jordan Rodgers. You are…"

In return, he extends his hand out to connect with mine for a proper handshake and says, "I'm Alfonzo Brown. It's nice to meet you."

"So, Mr. Brown, what brings you out this way, if you don't mind me asking?"

With my peripheral view, I could see Destiny not too pleased with my question. At this point, I don't give a damn. This man is in the apartment that Destiny and I share, so I feel I have the right to ask him whatever I want. It's not like she told me the real reason why this man is having a meeting with us.

"Jordan, feel free to call me Alfonzo. I'm sure we're around the same age, so no need to call me by my last name. And to answer your, question I'm here to conduct business with you and Destiny."

"Hmmm! You have my full attention now. So what kind of business do you want to conduct?"

Alfonzo is shifting his eyes from me to Destiny as he continues to speak with professionalism as well as confidence in his voice. "I was highly impressed with the photos you took for my business card. In fact, I was so impressed that I have another business proposition that I think you will love."

With a sparkle in her eyes, Destiny delightfully nods her head and smiles like she was agreeing with the business proposal before it was properly presented.

"Thank you. I take pride in everything I do, especially photography."

"Indeed you do. Your work speaks volumes about how much pride and expertise you have in photography. So much that I would love for you to take the photos for the cover of my book of poems that I've wrote over the years. Of course, I want no one other than you to take my photo to be placed on the back cover of my first book of poems."

"As soon as you send a copy of a contract to my lawyer and once he says everything is legit with the contract agreement, then I would be more than elated to work with you again."

"Great. I already have your lawyer information, so I will send a copy of the contract over to him first thing in the morning."

Destiny, at this point, is so excited I would think she's about to pee in her panties. How she is dancing around, shifting her weight from one leg to another. Besides her being overjoyed, I think I remember where I saw Alfonzo at. It was at the Poetry Club. When he said something about a book of poems he wrote, I connected the dots. This man seems to be strictly about his business. He's a true example of a workaholic.

"Now I have something to share with you that will make you happy, Jordan," he says as he turns his eyes toward me.

"Is that right?" I say with a hint of inquisitiveness.

"Yes. Destiny told me you're an entrepreneur as well. I've heard you want to open a bar down in Atlanta, Georgia, right?"

"Well, it's good to know that she hasn't told you all bad things about me. Anyway, you're very correct about that. My best friend and I are working on picking out a location for our sports bar. Location and getting a great interest rate on a loan from the bank seem to be our biggest challenge."

"When starting any business, location is always important. It's just important as having the money to start the business…I suppose."

With my eyebrow raised, I look at him with a desire to know what he got to say that will make me elated.

"Umm…so tell me more about what's supposed to make me happy."

"Well, let me not keep you guessing any longer," he says with a slight smile. "I work for Rich Finance, and I'm sure you know that we're a finance company that offers loans to students and first-time business owners and small-business owners. Destiny told me about how you and your business partner been looking for a decent interest rate that will fit in your budget. I do believe we can negotiate an interest rate that will work perfectly for the both of us."

Finding it difficult to hide the excitement in my voice, I somehow open my mouth and speak without revealing how I truly feel about the effects this conversation is having on me.

"I'm listening…"

"Of course, we have to do a credit check, but before the company runs a credit report, we can guarantee that the interest rate can be a minimum of fifteen percent, depending how excellent your credit is. So how much money do you think you will need to start your business?"

"This deal sounds more fascinating than butt-naked stripper on a pole."

Out the corner of my eye, I can see Destiny shaking her head in deep disgust. I get a feeling that I will hear about this later when Alfonzo leaves. As soon as he leaves, there may be another love and war going on…possibly just a war going on between us, without the love factor.

"My partner and I suggest that anywhere from fifty to seventy thousand dollars will be more than enough money to start our business."

I watch as he wrote the figures down for future reference. He seems to take his job very seriously. He seems to know when to have fun and when it's time for business. He certainly makes that transition look easier said than done. I may be able to learn a few things from him.

"I look forward to doing business with you, Jordan. I promise the both of you that you will hear from me within the next couple of days. If I have any more questions, I will contact you, Jordan, and feel free to contact me if you have any other questions or concerns."

As we shake hands and say our good-byes, I feel more than eager to share the good news with Markus. He will love to hear that we're close to getting a bank to approve us for the business loan we want with a low interest rate. As soon as Alfonzo leaves, I'll hit Markus up on his cell to inform him.

SHAPING UP

My business life seems to be shaping up nicely. There were times when I didn't know if Markus and I could really become big-time entrepreneurs. Our senior year in high school, we set a goal for ourselves that we would go to college for a business administration so we can be the best entrepreneurs we can be. He wanted to open up a poetry spot similar to the one he performs at. I wanted to open a strip club. For a long time we went back and forth about why our idea was better than the other. I would say, "Atlanta is home of the strip club, so why not open up a strip club? That's where the money is.

He would always say, "No, we need to enlighten our young brothers and sisters through deep, empowering messages that give them food for thought."

Markus always has been Afro-centric. He always has been an old soul as well. There is no doubt about it; Markus absolutely loves his black people. Not to confuse Markus as the racist type; he only wants to see his African American people reach and earn success. When we got tired of debating about our business aspirations, we decided on a sports bar. I'm more into basketball while he's more into football. The common ground was, we both love sports even though we like some sports more than the other. I came up with the name of the sports bar, Gear Up Sports Bar & Grill, while we both brainstormed about the vision of our business.

Seconds after Alfonzo left, I pick up my phone off the charger to call my boy. After a few rings, Markus answers the phone. "Wait, woman, let me answer the phone. What going on, bruh?" he says while trying desperately to hide the pleasure in his voice.

"Umm, I should be asking you that question," I say as I continue to hear slurping coming from his end. I already know that Asia and Markus are some big-ass freaks. Those to newlyweds can't seem to keep their hands off each other. I can hear in his voice that Markus is having a hard time keeping his composure on the phone.

"I'm going call you back in ten minutes," Markus somehow manages to say before hanging up abruptly.

Damn, I didn't even get a chance to say nothing else before he hung up. I guess I could give him a pass this time for the rude exit off the phone. I mean, it did sound like he was receiving some sexual healing.

About twenty minutes later, Markus finally decides to call back. The adrenaline rush from receiving what seems like the best news of my life at this moment has me impatiently waiting for my cell to ring. That's the real reason why I was overzealously watching the time like an underpaid worker ready to get off work.

Answering the phone without saying hello, I say, "It's about damn time you call a nigga back. Asia got ya ass pussy whipped."

"Naw, boy, you got it all wrong—we both whipped," he says with laugher in his voice.

Only I could say something like that to Markus without him thinking I am being derogatory about his marriage. We know each other's sense of humor as well as how far to push it.

"You already in a good mood, but I have something that will place you in an even better mood. Destiny brought by one of her clients who works in finance. He goes by the name of Alfonzo Brown, and he wants to do business with us. He's guaranteeing that he can offer us a loan with low interest rates so we can jump-start our business."

"Oh, for real…" Markus says in disbelief.

"Yes, I'm serious, nigga. He said that he works for a company called Rich Finance. He's promising low interest rates, depending on how good our credit is. In a couple days, he's going reach back out to me. If we need to reach him before then, we can call him."

"I'm trying not to get overexcited just yet because I will need to do my own research on Rich Finance. I've never heard of the company before, so I'm assuming it's a Detroit-based company."

Markus always analyzes a situation until he feels comfortable enough to follow through with a plan. He's never to act too quick off emotion to the point of making impulsive decisions. I'm happy I have a business partner like him, because if it were up to me, I wouldn't do any research on Rich Finance. In a situation like this, I would've acted off emotion.

"You know what, I didn't think to ask him if Rich Finance is all over the States. I was so caught in the business proposition that he presented."

"If I didn't know how to keep my composure when conducting business, we would be filing for bankruptcy," Markus says with a deep sigh of frustration.

"You know I'm overzealous about getting our business off the ground, so anytime an offer that sounds good is on the table, I get overexcited."

"I never automatically think someone is legit after one meeting. I have to read contracts and do research on the company before I get deeply involved."

I sit through about ten more minutes of Markus lecturing me about conducting business properly before we both get off the phone. Although Markus wasn't letting much of his emotion show, I know he was just as ecstatic as I am. We dreamed about being an entrepreneur for a while now.

Today may have started out a li'l rocky for me, but now it's coming along smooth. I want to just keep the momentum going with the good energy. Tonight I wish I could celebrate Density's and my accomplishments with Markus and Asia. What with our achieving this far within a year of graduation is amazing. Although physically Markus and Asia aren't here to celebrate with us tonight, I can still feel their energy. I know those two well, so I already know that if they were here, how turned up they would be.

Tonight my baby and I are going out for dinner and then going to her favorite reggae spot. I'm more into hip-hop and R&B than reggae, but I can tolerate it sometimes. Destiny's taste in music is a lot more versatile than mine. As well as how she chooses her friends. Our neighbor is sweeter than Now & Later and Jolly Ranchers put together, but of course, Destiny clicks with him without a problem. Stereotypically I always thought a woman will always have at least one gay male friend. It always seems that gay men who are super flamboyant always flock to girly girls. My assumption is they flock to them because they want to be women, and of course, they can't relate to straight man.

My mom befriended a couple of gay men. She claims that the bonhomie of their spirit is beautiful. When I ask whether she thinks it's right for two men to be sleeping together, she always says that "he who has not sin may cast the first stone." Unlike other Christians, my mom practices what she preaches. As long as I can remember, she treats everyone equally. I never hated or physically harmed a faggot, but I always feel uncomfortable being around them. I just want to look them in the eyes and tell them to "man the fuck up. You have a dick between your legs, not a pussy."

As we gather our things to get ready for our date, of course, we run into our neighbor. With his eyebrows looking like they were drawn on his face from getting arched and with his lip gloss popping, it would probably make any straight man uncomfortable. He always seems friendly, but I can't see myself saying hey and bye to him. We have nothing in common. Our lifestyles are and always will be totally different. Besides, I don't want people to think I'm on the down low. There's nothing DL about me. I want a woman, someone who can take my seed and sprout out a baby boy or girl. Like usual, I will allow the two of them to chat while I walk to the car, not going to let an awkward moment ruin my night. I will make sure tonight's going end in wonderful bliss.

PLAN OF ACTION IN MOTION

Last week was a highlight of my life. The business meeting between Alfonzo, Destiny, and me went so well. Surprisingly, Destiny and I got along all week after hearing such good news that could jump-start our careers. Unfortunately, Alfonzo wasn't able to schedule a second business meeting within a couple days like he promised. Now that I had left work at the Lefty's Lounge, I'm heading over to Rich Finance, where Alfonzo works. Lefty's Lounge is in midtown, as well as Rich Finance, so it won't be a long drive. I usually work a full shift during the day, crossing over until the night, because at night, that's when I make my tips. Alcoholics tend to come out at night, especially on the weekends. I love being a bartender because I get to learn more about what it takes to establish a successful sports bar.

    Not even traffic could slow down the scintilla of excitement I'm feeling right now. Riding to my destination with my AC on chill, I listen to Mary J. Blige's "Family Affair." I just love the production Dr. Dre did on this track. This shows Dr. Dre and Mary's versatility as music artists. As a businessman, I want to show this much versatility. As a future entrepreneur, I want my hands in many investments that will guarantee a major profit in the long run. Never been the type of guy to hustle by selling dope. However, I always have been a hustler who aimed to be the best I can be when it comes to getting the money or gaining recognition for work I do. I'm more like Jay-Z or Diddy, as opposed to Tony Montana. I hustle, but it's a different type of hustle game I'm in.

As I pull up in the park deck, I glance at the time. I've made it here in perfect time. Markus should be calling me at any second to confirm that he's ready for our video conference. Since Markus can't be here, we all agreed that we will have a video conference so we both can be informed about the business aspects.

Walking up to the building, I can't lie I'm feeling a slight bit insecure. Everyone around me is walking around with a suit and tie with a briefcase in their hands. Here I am, dressed way too casual for a meeting that could be pivotal to starting my entrepreneurship. Markus's ass is going to be on camera, looking *GQ* and shit, while I'm looking like I just walked off the pages of *Source* magazine. Today I'm going take a page out of Markus's book. Fuck what anyone thinks of my ensemble. I'm just as educated as any mothafucka in this building. The elevator opens up, then suddenly my phone starts ringing. Without looking, I know exactly who it is.

"Damn! I thought you forgot about the meeting for a second. I had expected you to call sooner than this," I say as I open the door that has gold writing stamped across it that read Rich Finance.

"I know right. I was expecting to call sooner but had to run a few errands before calling you. I'm at home now. I'm set and ready to go," Markus says.

While continuing to have small talk with Markus, I am taking in the exquisite scenery of the office. I expect it to be just a plain office building with simple décor that anyone could conjure up. The way the office of Rich Finance is set up lives up to every bit of its name. The cherry oak tables in the lobby across from the receptionist's desk have crystal decorations. Some chairs are the color of coffee with cream while the others are a milk-chocolate color. Anywhere the eye could see, the name of the company or logo imprinted on anything is always engraved in gold. The receptionist desk is made of glass with gold trimming. Astonishingly, even the receptionist has a really nice view of the city. I must say, this company is living up to its name. I'm beyond curious to know how Alfonzo's office looks like.

Walking up to the receptionist, suddenly a man appears, dressed professionally with a bowtie. Oh boy, he is dressed like Fonzworth Bentley. Everyone who follows hip-hop knows that Fonzworth Bentley is classic for wearing a bowtie. I am somewhat surprised it is a man at the receptionist's desk. I assumed that it would be a woman. My opinion is this is a woman's job, not a man's. You can call me sexist, but that's just how I feel about it.

"I'm here to see Alfonzo Brown for a 2:30 appointment," I say after placing Markus's on hold momentarily.

"Okay, sir. Will you just sign the list in front of you and Mr. Brown will be with you shortly. Let me know if you need any more assistance," he says with a smile.

"Okay, thank you."

The guy looks like he works out at the gym on a regular basis, so why the hell would he be doing a woman's job? Like my homie Markus, he's very brawny. Although he's shorter than Markus, he seems to be very physically fit, like a trainer. I don't know; maybe he's just sitting in for someone who couldn't make it today.

A few short minutes later, the guy behind the glass desk tells me that Alfonzo is ready for me. I hang up the phone with my homie as he leads me down the hall. After a couple of knocks on the door, I hear a tense voice say, "Come in." I could imagine how stressed he could be. The fact he's a young man working in an established finance company while trying to prove himself must feel like a burden sometimes.

Magically, the tension in voice was effaced once we came in the room. I'm not sure how. Alfonzo smiles at the man in front of me once he entered the room, and he smiles back.

"Thank you, Byron," Alfonzo says.

Hmm, I wonder what that was about. There must be some inside joke I don't know about. Whatever it was, about I don't care, because it's time to talk about business. Whatever distinctive languages those two are passing to each other in code, it is between them.

"Hey, man. How are ya?" I say while giving him a firm handshake.

"I'm just fine so far, it's been a long day. So how does Markus wish to participant in this meeting? Skype or ooVoo?" Alfonzo says with an elated look.

His office is spacious with a nice view of Motown. The office is neatly arranged with furniture, creative decorations, and paintings. The color scheme of his décor is mostly earth-tone color with a smudge of gold. I assume that his color scheme must fit his personality, but then again, I'm not sure since I don't know much about him.

"Skype. His username is Seasoned_Soul."

"His name sounds familiar. I remember a poet that went by the name Seasoned. I believe I heard his spoken word for the first time at the Poetry Club down in my home city of Atlanta."

"Right. I thought I've seen you at the Poetry Club before. It dawned on me where I saw you after you mentioned you're putting together a book of poetry. And yes, Markus's stage name is Seasoned."

"If we are talking about the same guy, I love Seasoned's spoken word he entitled 'The Struggle.'"

"Yes, we're talking about the same guy. 'The Struggle' had a powerful message attached to it as well as a strong delivery. I remember that night. I believe you had some words on the subject of equality that night. It made me really think about how things would be if we all were truly treated equal."

"All right, let's not get distracted by poetry," Alfonzo says with a slight grin as he continues to speak. "I want to get back to the subject that matters right now, and that's to put some money in your account to start your business. We can definitely get together some other time and chat more about poetry."

"I will take you up on that offer."

Comfortably I sit back in the chair across from Alfonzo's stylish desk and wait for him to log on to Skype to video-chat with Markus. Within a few short minutes of silence, Alfonzo informs me that he had found Markus's username on Skype. In just a few seconds, or perhaps minutes, an essential moment that I will never forget is about to occur. When getting out your dreams, you got to have a plan. Without a plan of action and doing what it takes to make your dreams come true, you won't succeed. For the first time in this process of working on becoming an entrepreneur, I feel that I'm making the right steps in the right directions. My intuition tells me that I'm where I need to be.

"Hey, Jordan, I don't mean to break you out your daydream, but I have Markus on Skype. If you would like, you can pull your chair around on the side of the desk so he can see both of us while we discuss this," Alfonzo says with a slight chuckle.

"My bad. I was slightly in a daydream," I say as I pull my chair over to the side of the desk.

Just like I predicted, Markus is dressed up like he was getting ready to pose for *GQ* magazine. My homie has on a gray-and-purple striped button-down shirt along with a slim gray tie. To bring the look all together, he has on a white vest. Our styles are so different, but we are great business partners as well as friends. He made the room I was sleeping in when we were roommates his own personal office, so I already knew that's where he's sitting at right now.

"It's nice to finally meet you, Markus. Your business partner has told me about the plans you both have for each other's future. The pleasure is mine to be the one to conduct business with the both of you here at Rich Finance."

"It's nice to meet you as well, Alfonzo. I appreciate you giving us the opportunity to even discuss business with you. We've been working diligently on getting the ball rolling since we graduated from Clark Atlanta University."

"What a small world. I graduated from Clark Atlanta last year as well. Although, I don't remember seeing you or Jordan on campus. I guess each of us ran in different social groups."

"Right. I do believe that we did, because I don't recall seeing you on campus. I do remember you from the Poetry Club. Maybe we can collaborate on something when you're back in town, but in the meantime, let's discuss more about this business loan, if you don't mind," Markus says with a slight aggression, changing the subject to what matters the most.

Markus isn't trying to be rude, but just like Alfonzo, he's strictly about the business. If he ain't doing nothing to better himself, especially when it comes to his personal life, he ain't going to be involved. This meeting is the pivotal point of his career, so he's not going take this for granted. Neither am I.

"Awww…yes. We checked the credit of the both of you and happy to inform that y'all are approved for up to a sixty-thousand-dollar loan. Your interest rate will be fifteen percent for the course of ten-year period."

"If we choose a longer payment term, will that affect our interest rate going up?" I ask.

"Yes, say if you want a twenty-year period, then your interest rate will go up ten percent because of the extent of years added on the agreement."

"Everything sounds good so far. Will you fax a copy of everything written in paper so I can look over the agreement you're offering us," says Markus.

"I sure will once you give me your fax number, and I will send it right over to you. Jordan, I can give you a copy of everything in black and white, so you can look over it if you want. I don't expect anyone to sign without further discretion."

"Thanks. I will truly appreciate that."

Overall, the meeting went very well. The offer that Alfonzo presented to us was the best offer we had thus far. Tonight, I have to do something special for Destiny because if it weren't for her, we would've never met Alfonzo.

Leaving the offices of Rich Finances, I feel like I was walking on air. The feeling I have is amazingly intangible. No one, or nothing, can bring me down. I'm so happy at the moment. Our plans are finally in motion as soon as if we look a few things over.

THE BREAKUP

Looking down at my phone, I notice it's only 3:30 in the afternoon. I am feeling overjoyed after the meeting went so well. It's a good thing I had told my boss I was taking the rest of the day off. My intuition tells me that everything would be fine during the meeting. I had faith that God would work things out in our favor about starting our business I just needed to test my faith more.

On the way home, I'm going to buy Destiny's favorite wine so we can celebrate. When she gets home, a bubble bath will be waiting to hug her every curve while she sinks into what will seem like a never-ending relaxing sensation.

Halfway home after leaving the liquor store, my phone starts to ring. Turning the music down, I answer it, and before I could say hello, Markus just starts talking loudly in my ear.

"We on our way, baby!"

"Got damn! Calm your ass down. You loud as fuck in my ear," I say in a playful way.

"I looked over the paperwork, and everything seems legit. I'm faxing a copy over to our business lawyer now so he can make sure there's no malicious fine print that we don't know about."

"I couldn't tell on Skype if you gave a damn or not. You good at keeping your composure no matter what happens for as long as I've known you. Well, most of the time, because I do remember the Quinesha incident."

"I have to stay professional no matter how excited I may be. Of course I will smile or shake my head in agreement when I hear something I like, but for the most part, I keep all my exhilaration to myself until it's time to turn up. And usually I keep my cool pretty well unless provoked. You know that, bruh."

"You're right. I know how you are. So what you going to do to celebrate?"

"I'm not sure, but I want you to personally tell Destiny that I appreciate her introducing you to Alfonzo and looking out for us. We probably would've never got a great deal offer if it weren't for her playing an important role in just introducing us to the right people."

"Yeah, man. I'm going to make sure I let her know how grateful you are. I'm going to show my gratitude tonight when she comes home from a photo shoot."

"Maybe you should reach out to your parents. I'm sure they will love to hear the good news about getting a business loan offer."

"Naw, I'm not in the mood to speak to either one of them today. I will call my mama soon though. On second thought, I have a great idea as far as promoting our sports bar. You know my cousin is a well-known DJ in Atlanta, so it won't be difficult for him to shout our spot out on the radio."

"That's a good idea. The more free publicity, the better. I'll let you get home, and we got to talk again soon because I think I found a place right outside of the Buckhead area. Technically it will still be considered DeKalb County instead of Fulton but will be broader line to Fulton County, which would make our bar be in Atlanta without the expensive prices of owning a business in the heart of the city."

"Wow…that's a blessing. I never thought about looking for a location that's broader line to Fulton County. We could definitely capitalize on being in such a great location. Keep me posted."

God is truly blessing me. He must be listening to my prayers, or either my mama still praying for me. Either way, things are looking up for me. I probably should listen to Markus and call my mama. It would be good to hear her voice. This has to be the longest grudge I held against my mama. It's ordinary for me not to speak or hear from Samuel for long periods at a time. Not hearing from that deadbeat doesn't bother me one bit. Hopefully, soon all the burdens dealing with my parents can be laid down to rest. Then I can finally feel like I don't have anything to prove to myself or Samuel that I'm nothing like him.

Getting out my car with Destiny's favorite bottle of wine in a brown paper bag, I walk up the steps to our apartment. As I approach my apartment, my eyes witness something that made me feel abruptly saturated in sick. My neighbor and his boyfriend are kissing before they walk in their apartment. They are pulling at each other's clothes right before they close the door. Those niggas are acting like they're the only people in the world. They could've done all that nasty shit behind closed doors. I didn't ask to witness that. One thing I must admit; they're confident with their sexuality, but I suppose they're too confident. They don't have a problem bringing what they do in the dark into the light.

I walk on to my place. As I unlock the door and turn the key, I am still shaking that intense vision out of my mind. No time to waste now because Destiny will be home soon, but not before I finish cooking some spaghetti with meatballs. I place on a slow mix to set the mood as I prepare dinner. We both made a few mix CDs that cater to both of our tastes. Destiny likes the up-to-date slow jams as well as some '90s music. Meanwhile, I'm a fan of the '80s and '90s slow jams more than the new stuff that's out now. I want things to be perfect from the time she walks through the door until the time we wake up in each other's arms tomorrow morning.

Grabbing my cell, I text my baby to see what time she will be coming home so I will know what kind of time constraint I'm facing. Shortly after sending the texted, she texts back, letting me know she will be home in thirty minutes. The meal is almost ready. I plan on starting the bubble bath five minutes prior to the time she's supposed to arrive because I know it's going be an additional ten minutes before she actually arrives. When she walks through the door, I will have one of her favorite songs playing: "Loving Me 4 Me" by Christina Aguilera. I know hearing one of her favorite songs playing as she walks through the door while the aroma of food hitting her nose will set her in a romantic mood.

I have the bubble bath ready while the candles burn slowly near the tub, leaving an imprint of mandarin tangerine scents at every corner of the room. Tonight I'm showering her with her favorites—favorite scented candles along with her favorite way to relax.

Making my way back to kitchen, I hear keys fumbling, so I know it must be her at the door. With the remote to the surround sound in my hand, I quickly skipped to number 1 on the CD. As she fumbles with the key, I position myself halfway in the living room, facing the door with my shirt off, revealing abs that I worked so hard for back in college. As stand there facing the door waiting for Destiny to open the door, I hold two wineglasses in my hand with a huge smile on my face. Destiny loves to see me with my shirt off, revealing the few tats I have on my chest. My abs and chest were how I caught her attention years ago in college. My goal is to make sure I get a whole lot of her attention tonight, not only in the bedroom, but also the bathroom, the kitchen counter, making our way down to the floor.

As I watch the key turn the lock to the right, I know it is almost time for lights, camera, action. The door swings open at what seems like five miles per hour. Suddenly I notice Destiny has some bags in her hands. My eyes get big that it isn't designer clothes from the mall, instead it is bags with groceries in them. The fact that she came in without one bag from the mall is flabbergasting to me. I set the wineglasses down on the nearest coffee table so I could help with the bags. While grabbing some of the bags from her hands, I kick the door shut with my foot.

"Welcome home, babe. I prepared dinner and a bubble bath for you to show my appreciation for you," I say as we walk toward the kitchen together.

"That's nice of you. Once I put the groceries away, I think I'll take a bath and relax. After I'm done, we need to talk," she says, looking distraught.

"What's wrong? Did something happen at work?"

"No, nothing happened at work. We can talk about it lata, once I finish bathing."

Without waiting for another word, she rushes right past me toward our room. Even if I was in the mood to argue, I would have to run behind her to state my case. Maybe she's on her period or something, because we haven't had a disagreement in a long time. Usually our disagreements come when I mention kids and then she brings up marriage. Those topics haven't been discussed between us lately since the day I met Alfonzo for the first time. While she calms down, I'm just going to focus on setting the table. Once she gets done prepping after her bath, she may be ready to have a more settled romantic evening for two.

As the music continues to play softly in the background, sending falsetto vocals of Prince's "Scandalous" throughout our place, I hum along. It's as if the bells of the intro of the song called Destiny out, because simultaneously, she comes into the view a few feet from the dining table. I had a bowl of salad on the table, set with two plates of spaghetti. There she is, standing in front of me in an oversized shirt of mine with her hair hanging freely. No makeup and she's still flawless to me. My mind's suddenly corrupted by libidinous thoughts of what she has on under my shirt. Nothing can ruin this night.

"Let me get your chair for you."

"You being really nice. What's the occasion?"

"I just want to say thank you for introducing me to Alfonzo, because thanks to you, Markus and I have the business loan we need to jump-start our business."

I smiled so hard as I spoke that you'd think I'm happy on something or slightly deranged. Making my way back to my seat once again, I notice Destiny seems to be in deep thought. It is kind of nagging at me because I spent all this time preparing a dinner for us and she sits across from me like she doesn't give a fuck.

"Is something wrong? Didn't you hear what I told you about the business loan?" I say as calmly as I can before taking a deep breath.

"I'm just going to be blunt. I appreciate everything you did for me tonight. I'm also happy for you and Markus. After long consideration, I think that we should pump the brakes on this relationship. I love you, but sometimes I feel like we need time to grow and figure out what we want to do in our personal lives, especially when it comes to business."

"What you mean figuring out what to do in our personal lives when it comes to business?"

"It's simple…you pressure me about children while I'm more career minded than raising a family so soon. I rather get married and be a power couple before starting a family. I'm not ready to be a mother."

"How long you been feeling like this?" I say with confusion and rage in my voice.

"You know I've been feeling like this, don't act dumb with me. I knew you would be upset with my decision, but since you playing clueless, I've been pondering this since our last big argument. You can stay here until you find somewhere else to go."

"Don't worry. I will be gone sooner than you think…matter of fact, I'm leaving now. So enjoy your dinner alone."

"Jordan, wait, don't be like that. I'm trying to do what's best. You know we need some time apart for a while."

Without listening to shit she had to say, I grab a few of my things, throw it in a gym bag, and head toward the door before putting on a shirt, feeling so fiery inside that all I could see is red. How this bitch going dump me after all these years? I moved my ass to Michigan to be with her high-maintenance ass, and this is the shit I have to put up with. I'm in my fuck-that-shit mood. I need to get in my car and drive.

THE BOND

As I cruise around the city of Motown, thinking to myself about everything that took place, I wonder whether I was stupid for moving all the way out here. Instead of putting my career first, I placed what I thought was best for our relationship first. I took it upon myself to move here in this cold-ass city back in January to be closer to her. We both knew our relationship wouldn't last with the long distance, especially once our careers started rolling. Now she's doing what maybe I should've done and told her I need some space to figure things out. I'm the fool for placing her before my career. Maybe I should call my mama. She may be able to give me some guidance on what to do. Then again she probably will say things I don't want to hear. I hear her now, "Maybe you should listen to why she feeling that way and express how you feel." I'm livid and not in the mood for some lecture from another woman. Women are always going to stick up for women in a situation like this. I'm sure.

    My love life is so dysfunctional that it has me discombobulated to the point I'm actually contemplating getting advice from Samuel. I know I'm out my mind now. Damn. At a time like this, it would be nice to get some support from my parents, but their relationship always has been dysfunctional as well. I figure that's why I'm the way I am now, because I never had much experience being around a tight family. My family isn't like the TV families where they sit around an open fire singing Christmas carols, eating gingerbread cookies. No picnics at the

Stone Mountain Park to see the fireworks on the Fourth of July. What do I know about parenting or building a stable relationship when all I ever saw was a relationship that constantly stood on shaky ground?

The world around me and everything in it seem to be irrelevant to me right now. Walking into the bar where I work, I'm sure they can tell I'm not myself. Shit, I didn't expect to come here. I was just driving, and before I knew it, I was here craving for a drink. The only thing that can quench my thirst is liquor. As I sit at the bar, anger must be written all over my face because none of my regular customers or coworkers speak to me. They must know it would be best to leave me alone as I continue to be in deep thought. In all honesty, I'm happy they didn't ask me what's wrong.

A few short minutes go by before I think I heard someone calling my name. It wasn't until I felt a large hand on my shoulder that I knew someone was indeed trying to get my attention. Fuck! I'm not in the mood to talk or listen to no one shit today. Why can't this mothafucka leave me alone like everyone else in this bitch? With one harsh look, I turn around to face the nigga who is disturbing me.

"Hey, man, I didn't know you were going be at work tonight. It seems like you have something on your mind that has you pugnacious. I'm down to listen if you want to vent," Alfonzo said with concern written all over his face.

Seeing how concerned he was and not only concerned but also serious about listening to me discuss my problems, I think maybe it wouldn't be a bad idea. I don't understand why he would care to listen since we barely even know each other. My mom always told me you don't have to know someone to help out a person who wants to be helped. At this moment, Alfonzo is proving to me that; my mama isn't the only one to think this way. A part of me certainly wants to be helped. Most of the time, when I'm filled with rage, it's against my jurisdiction to communicate with anyone, but this situation has me feeling a certain level of vulnerability.

"Destiny broke up with me. I packed a few of my things and left her ass at what used to be our home."

"I want to ask what caused her to make a decision, but where are you going stay now?"

"I was so upset with her decision to break up with me that I didn't think anything through. I instantly became impulsive. We had been getting along so well lately, so her stupid decision doesn't make sense to me."

"Maybe you should talk to her about how you feel once you cool down. I'm sure, with a clear head, you can hear her out and get the answer you need."

"Somewhere down the line I might consider doing that, but right now my pride won't allow me to let her know how much I'm hurting about the situation."

"I understand. Until you figure out where you going to go from here, I have an extra room in my apartment in Novi, so you're more than welcome to stay in my guest room until you get on your feet."

"Oh, naw, man, I don't want to burden you—"

"Naw, I insist you stay until you get back on your feet or work things out with Destiny. I know most of your family is back home in Georgia, so the least I can do is help out a man in need."

"I'm not a man in need, but I can admit you're right about everything else," I say in an offensive tone. "You're right about one thing though, all my family is back in Georgia."

Judging the tone in Alfonzo's voice, I can tell he mean well, so since I haven't thought everything through, it might be best to take him up on his offer. Since I moved here back in January, I haven't staked money in case something like this occurs. Now that Destiny slick kicked me out, I wish that I would've been smart enough to secretly stash away some money in case I need to find my own spot quick, fast, and in a hurry. It pains me to tell him that he's right about me being a man in need. I will not allow him to think I'm weak like I can't take care of myself. Slowly feeling my anger turn into pity, I just want to lie down to get some much-needed rest. With one nod of my head before taking my last shot to the head, I stumble out my chair on my feet to exit the bar.

"I don't think you need to be driving tonight since you've been drinking, so your best bet is to leave your vehicle here while you ride with me. I can, or Byron can, drop you off in the morning to pick up your car," says Alfonzo.

I can tell out my peripheral view that he is keeping an eye on me, making sure I wouldn't fall while walking in front of him toward the door. Little did he know that he didn't have to worry about me falling and busting my ass. I was concentrating on every step that I took. Not tonight will I be busting my ass in front everyone who is around to see.

What seem to be like only a few minutes later, we are at his residence. Novi is outside of Detroit, but with how fast Alfonzo drives, he made it seem like it's only few minutes away. Concentrating on my every step again, I slowly follow Alfonzo as he leads the way into his apartment. This is my first time coming to Novi, so if I'm going to be staying with Alfonzo for a while, I will have to learn my way around.

As I watch Alfonzo twist the doorknob and walk right in his apartment, I wonder whether the alcohol is playing tricks on me. That vodka must got me tripping, because I know this nigga didn't just walk in without using a key. Who leaves their door unlocked especially at night? Even if I'm packing some heat, I'm not going to leave the door to my crib unlocked. To my surprise, Byron, the guy who was working the receptionist desk, is sitting in the living room, watching the flat-screen TV as he if were expecting us. He must have seen us coming and left the door unlocked since the massive living room window gives a view to where we parked. We just so happened to park in front of the apartment. I'm slightly curious about why he's here and where he's sleeping if I'm going be in the guest room.

"I do believe you met Byron back at the office, Jordan. Never mind us, feel free to make yourself at home."

I nod my head in agreement that I remember him as I spoke to him, extending my hand to give him some dab.

"What up, Byron?"

"What up? Alfonzo told me that you would be coming over and staying in the guest room. I made sure that some fresh sheets were on the guest bed for you," Byron says.

"Thank you. Where is the guest room? I think I need to relax."

"It's down the hall on the right."

Walking down the hall, I admire for the first time the way the apartment is fixed up. When I walked through the door, I wasn't paying much attention to how nice the apartment is until now. Once again, Alfonzo's space is decorated with earth-tone colors. The colors in the living room expand from dark green with different shades of cream and brown. I'd never seen the color combination, but whoever decorated the room made it seem effortless. To set off the living room was a fifty-five-inch TV mounted on the wall. Judging on his taste, I'm sure it's a

LED smart TV. Not only does he have a nice television, he also has a nice-ass surround sound to go with it.

The living room kind of got me hyped to see what the guest room will look like. Entering the room, the first thing I notice is how clean and fresh it smells in here. Either someone keeps this room clean or Byron did a quick cleaning because he knew I was coming. The entire apartment seems to be spotless, so I would think they are extremely neat people. The bed has a black-and-white comforter on it with black and yellow pillows. Just a little more color than the living room with the yellow pillows. I have to ask him who fixed his place up. Whoever used their decorative skills to hook up his rooms, whomever he hired needs to hook up the rooms in my spot once I find one. She will be hired in a heartbeat for sure. I don't know shit about decorating a room, apartment, or office.

A knock at the door takes me away from admiration of the guest room, but not before I notice my own thirty-two-inch television mounted in front of the bed. Damn, Alfonzo must be ballin'.

"Come on in…door open."

"I came to bring you some fresh towels and rags. I'm sure you notice you have your own bathroom, so you don't have to wait until Byron or I finish in the bathroom, if you need to use it. Let me know if there's anything else I can do," Alfonzo says, standing in the doorway.

"Thanks. I must admit, you have a bad-ass apartment. You ballin'? Maybe I chose the wrong profession," I say with a slight chuckle.

"I appreciate that."

I watch him laugh for a bit while I think about asking for his opinion about my love life. I definitely can't call Markus or Uncle Joe up to get their opinion because it's late. They most likely will be asleep. What I want is another man's opinion.

"Can I ask you something?"

"Yes, I'm listening."

"One of the things Destiny and I would argue about was having kids. In fact, I know that's probably what pushed her to make a decision like she did. See, I want kids now, but she wants the ring and career before having children. Do you think I was pushing the issue too hard?"

"Before answering that question, I must ask what's the reason that you have such a peculiar desire to have kids?"

"You're right. My desire is somewhat distinctive. Most men my age are not thinking about marrying anyone or raising children. God knows I don't want to be engaged to anyone right now. However, God knows I would love to see my seed grow up to be the best man or woman he or she can be. The way I grew up without any siblings is part of why I feel the way I do. Plus my dad wasn't around all the time."

"I see…you should do some more soul-searching as to why you have this urge to have kids so soon. It seems to me that raising children is something that is important to you…like it will make you complete."

"I just want to prove to everyone who says I look like my dad that I'm nothing like him. I'm a better man than him. I will be a better father to my children than him. I will be there to see my children's first birthday, say their first words, and take their first steps."

"I don't think you pushed the issue too hard. Did you ever tell her all of this?"

"No."

"That's probably what you did wrong. Instead of telling her you want children, you should've told her why you feel this way. I'm sure these feelings you keep locked away is in a dark place, but sometimes it's okay to reveal your truth that lies in the dark. You can't keep your true feelings locked away forever. Like a tree without the light of the sun, it won't grow and spread its branches so the world can see its growth. Once you stop hiding your true emotions, that's when you start to shed light on your truth, and you and as well as others will start witnessing your growth."

With my ears and mind wide-open, I receive his words with total comprehension. The way he delivers his message to me isn't offensive but very profound. In all honesty, I do hide my demons, growing up without a stable father in my life, in complete darkness. If you don't know me, you wouldn't know that my fatherless past haunts me. The ghost of my past has latched on to me and, over the years, has been difficult for me to let go. For anyone who knows me will know that my fatherless past has affected me, but I do not like to shine light on it.

I've been tight with Markus for years. He's known me well enough to the point that he would never discuss how his dad taught him about safe sex or how to drive because he knew that would make me jealous. I always wanted the type of family Markus has. He has siblings that had the love from both parents. To this day, I can't remember his parents missing one of his football games. There were many times my mama couldn't make my basketball game because she had to work a double to provide for the both of us. She was my full-time parent who partnered with a part-time dad.

Life ain't fair for sure, so I need to work on letting go. Try and love again now that Samuel seems to have grown up. Ever since they renewed their vows, he moved back in as well as comes home from work every night. At least that's what my Aunt Bev told me the last time I spoke to her on the phone. It took Samuel twenty-two years to get his shit together. It's evident that he's changing for the better, so why can't I just forgive him?

Alfonzo has me evaluating myself as well as the decisions I made, not only in my relationship with Destiny, but with my parents as well. I slick feel like Alfonzo and I are bonding a li'l. Alfonzo was the missing puzzle piece that helped gel my business venture together. Now he's feeding me food for thought so profoundly. My mama told me time and time again that I need to forgive. I would hear her, but I wasn't listening to her. It's funny how sometimes you take advice from someone you barely know better than from someone whom you've known all your life.

Stripping back the covers as our conversation begins to end, my body waits anxiously to feel the comfort of this queen-sized pillow top. Alfonzo makes his way to the door as Byron walks by with a towel wrapped around his waist. I assume he's making his way to the shower before Alfonzo beats him to it.

"If you need to talk about anything, remember I'm willing to listen. I can't guarantee that I will have t-he perfect advice every time, but I'm here for you."

"Thanks, man."

"Talk to you in the morning. I'm about to take a shower and lay it down. I'm off tomorrow for the Fourth of July, but I will have no problem taking you to pick up your car."

"Anytime is fine because I took the Fourth off. Destiny and I have plans, but that's canceled now."

"Okay. Don't worry, everything will be fine."

Watching him go down the hall in the same direction as Byron, I continue with my thoughts now that I'm finally alone again. If there was a slight chance that growing up as a li'l boy you wouldn't be ridiculed for liking a certain color or liking R&B music, then maybe I could easily be more free expressing my feelings. Instead it seems like boys had to like the color blue plus listen to rap music or they would be considered soft. After years of hiding anything that makes me feel defenseless, I don't seem to know how to do anything else. Alfonzo's lines from his equality poem echoes in my head.

> *Living in today's society, there's a new meaning to R. Kelly's "down low." Living in today's society, women can do some things in the light what others have to do in the dark.*

Those lines have a meaning to me now. At first I was trying desperately to figure out what he meant. Someday I will ask him about that poem. At this moment, it means to me that women have more free will to openly share their temperaments while men hide their feelings in the dark on the low. The meaning of his lines will probably be different from mine; however, this is my own interpretation of what it means to me.

EQUALITY

The smell of bacon floats its way through the air, creeping silently under the door as the sun peaks through the binds. The scent of the wavy piece of pork has my stomach singing praises to God for allowing me to see another day. The only thing I can think about now is eating some blueberry waffles. Anytime I eat bacon, I love to have some blueberry waffles with some cheese and eggs. Today some plain waffles will do. I'm not big on eating breakfast every morning. A bowl of cereal is good enough for me to start my day. Destiny or my mama never could figure out why I never was crazy about eating a huge breakfast in the morning as much as I love to eat. The both of them love to eat a healthy breakfast every morning.

Destiny can be stubborn sometimes, but she always did know how to take care of me. Prior to living together, she would occasionally cook me breakfast. If I wasn't over her place, she would bring the food over to my dorm. Whenever, for some reason she didn't cook, she would even take me out to IHOP or the Waffle House. She would make sure I would at least have a good meal before my first morning class. Envisioning her in the kitchen now in my T-shirt and some panties, fixing everything that I like, makes me miss her more and more. One day I will have to exploit my feelings. Then she will understand how I think. Then she will understand why I push so hard to have a child. Like people say, I will have to cross that bridge when the time comes. As of right now, I just want to do what I do every morning, which is brush my teeth, shower, and wash my face before going to the kitchen, where the food is.

This will be my first time walking into the kitchen. However, I do trust and believe that it will be an easy find. I'm just going to let my nose direct me to where I need to be. I walk up the hall toward the front door. As I get closer the front door, I made a left toward the kitchen. Byron and Alfonzo are at the dining table but aren't saying a word. That's how I know the food must be damn good. As I walk closer to the table, Byron makes eye contact with me first.

"I knew my nose wouldn't deceive me. This nice breakfast woke me up out my sleep. I couldn't let y'all have all the food," I say with a laugh.

"Naw, that wouldn't be right to leave our guest without a decent breakfast while we in here chowing down," Byron says sarcastically before continuing on to say, "We even have a plate ready for you."

Alfonzo doesn't say anything, just kept right on eating his meal with a smile on his face as he listens to Byron and me talk briefly. Admiring what's supposed to be my plate, I couldn't help but lick my lips. Two waffles, bacon, and some eggs with a tall glass of orange juice are waiting for my arrival. Byron gets up from the table immediately after eating to wash the dishes. He seems to know his way around the kitchen pretty well as he has been living here for a while. My guess is the two of them have been roommates for a while.

"How long you and Byron been roommates?"

Looking up from his almost-empty plate, Alfonzo looks up at me with a crease going across his forehead. He must be thinking about how long they been living together, I suppose. Byron turns around to look at Alfonzo with his arms crossed, as if he better say the right thing. In all honesty, that seems like something Destiny would've done if someone asked me how long we'd been dating. Nevertheless, I know that in this case, Alfonzo can't be homo, because I know a faggot when I see one. Alfonzo doesn't act nothing like the punks who live next door to Destiny. There's no "Hey, boo" or "Hey, gurl, honey, chile" in his vernacular; if so, that would be definitely be a gay behavior.

"For about six weeks," Alfonzo says before looking over at Byron with a smirk on his face. "Naw...I was joking, we've been living together for a year."

"I can tell, he knows his way around the kitchen pretty well."

"If I get in the kitchen, the whole apartment will be burned down with everything in it."

In unison we all laugh our ass off while Byron laughs the most like he could picture the whole scene. These two seem to get along well. I'm not sure what the meaning of their friendship is, but they seem to have a mutual brotherly bond between each other. Although sometimes it do seem kind of weird how they act around each other. I just know when I was roommates with Markus, I never cooked for him and then wash the dishes.

"I'm about to make some business calls in the bedroom for our party tonight after cleaning the kitchen. Jordan, if you don't have anything planned, you should come, but you have to leave a close mind at the front door if you come out," Bryon says after wiping a tear away from the corner of his eye from laughing so hard.

"Once Alfonzo takes me to my car, I'm going to stop by Destiny's place and try to talk. Where's the party going to be at?"

"Actually, it's going be at Alfonzo's and my club. The party starts at ten."

"Oh, I didn't know y'all invested in a club. What you mean leave a close mind at the front door," I say with one eyebrow raised.

"We opened up Club Liberal a few months ago. I wanted to open up a club where anyone can come and be who they are. I knew that in order for me to get out my dream, I had to get a business loan as well as become a connoisseur of running a nightclub. After doing my homework, I went into Rich Finance to apply for a business loan, and that's how I met Alfonzo. Not only did I get approved for a loan, but I also found a job within the company."

I switch my attention to Alfonzo as he stands and walks over to Byron to place his arm around his shoulder while he emphasizes more about everything. Meanwhile, I'm patiently waiting on my question to be answered.

"Just like you and Markus, Byron gave me a business pitch about what his dreams were. Within no more than five minutes, I was a believer that the idea could make not only him some money but me as well. You know by now that I'm all about making a smart investment, so I partnered with Byron on this business venture."

"So basically the target crowd is everyone no matter age or gender?"

"Yes," says the both of them.

"Each night is geared toward specific age groups. For example, Friday nights is for the eighteen and up partygoers. On Friday nights, the DJ will play mostly hip-hop and some R&B, meanwhile Saturday night is for the grown and sexy. No one can enter if they are younger than twenty-five. On Saturday night, the DJ will play mostly R&B music."

"So is this why you say 'leave a close mind at the front door'?"

Byron and Alfonzo both look at each other with slight uneasiness, as if I were placing ten tons of duress on their shoulders. To me, I look at it as a simple question. If Byron felt uncomfortable or didn't know how to answer, the question he should've not made the statement he made.

"Let's just put it this way...the name of the club speaks for itself. We simply named the club Liberal because we want people to lay their burdens down before walking into the club. Out in today's society, people may have a hard time being who they want to be. They may have a difficult time being free. When a customer walks into our spot, we want them to feel like they're behind closed doors. So if someone has a closed mind, they will not feel comfortable at our club," says Alfonzo.

Alfonzo seems to be always preaching equality. Now would be the best time to ask him about his spoken word at the Poetry Club last year. Last night I gather my own interruption of what he meant. Now I want to know exactly what he may have meant.

"All this talk about liberation reminds me of your equality poem. You know, the one where you refer to down low having a different meaning now..."

Before I could complete my sentence, he has started allowing the lines that stood out to me roll right off his tongue, so smooth like water flowing down a stream. I watch in amusement as he leaves Byron's side, making his way toward the table, eyes glued on me like he was auditioning for a movie role. Whenever he speaks those words, it seems to make him reminisce about something in his past, I assume. The passion in his tone makes him embody vulnerability like it was his fashion sense.

"Living in today's society, there's a new meaning to R. Kelly's 'down low.' Living in today's society, women can do some things in the light what others have to do in the dark."

"Wow! That was more dynamic than the first time I heard you say it."

"As a man, we are taught differently than a woman. There are stereotypes that both men and women of all color have to do with. For example, some of men's individualities our based on when he lost his virginity or how many numbers he got at the mall, because as people say, boys are going to be boys. On the other hand, if a woman thinks that way, they're more so labeled a hoe. Not saying that men have it easy by all means. We may get the pass to give the dick to every woman with a pulse but easily get criticized if we show any tendencies of doing the opposite. I do believe that's why so many men are on the low about their sexuality, because they were taught it's wrong to be aroused by the same sex. On the other hand, women have the free will to walk around in the day of light expressing their sexuality."

"That makes a lot of sense. I'm sure there are millions of men in the world who aren't gay or in the closet that still have a hard time dealing with their emotions."

"The poem I wrote isn't about homosexuality in general, instead it's about broken barriers that men can't be treated equal just because they show vulnerability. Men have feelings just like women, do not matter how tough they are or how they choose to cover it up. I have lesbian, gay, and straight friends that had an incident relating to this topic. Hell, even I had some issues with expressing myself because I was afraid I would be looked at as soft."

With Alfonzo breaking down his inspiration behind his equality poem, it has helped me see the fault in myself. I can't speak for every man; however, I can speak for myself. Throughout my life I was used to being tough or having sex with different girls as a defense mechanism. The thing is, my definition of being tough has been to never let another human being see you cry, when in actuality, the tough individuals are the men who don't give a damn about who see them cry. The one who is really tough is the man who can stay monogamous throughout the course of a relationship without giving a damn if another man thinks he's pussy whipped.

WE CRY TOGETHER

On the way from Novi to downtown Detroit, I sit on the passenger side of Alfonzo's car, not saying much. No disrespect toward Alfonzo, but I think he could read my body language well because he didn't bother me this time. After discussing everything with him last night, he knows that I need time to think. I seem to clear my head the most when I'm driving my own car with the music of my choice playing softly. Particularly something that's soulful with a self-conscious message. As of now, riding on the passenger side as random songs come on the radio will have to do.

    Communicating with Alfonzo about my own issues has taken a load off my chest. He has clearly helped shine some light on flaws that I have within me that I didn't want anyone to see. With a different outlook on whether I should open up about expressing my sentiments to Destiny or not, now I believe we can have a civilized conversation. Now is the time. There won't be no screaming at each other like we're out in the jungle, acting like wild animals. A lack of communication along with showing that I have listening skills is what's been missing in our relationship. If we can't see eye-to-eye, how are we gonna bring a child into this world? Conceiving a child with Destiny right now will make me feel like a failure.

    Now I realize that if we had a baby before the both of us are ready, I will be making the same mistake as Samuel. Then I will ask myself how having a baby before I'm ready will prove that I'm a better man than him if I'm making the same mistake as he did twenty-two years ago. All these years I've worked at convincing myself that I'm ready to have children; now I can honestly say that I'm not. The day my son or daughter is born, I need to know that I'm ready to show my seed what it takes to be a strong person. I'm just beginning to learn that valuable lesson the hard way. Destiny was right; I need to focus on my career. I have my whole life ahead of me to reproduce as many representations of me as I want. Every child that my woman bears is going to be a piece of me. They will represent me and my last name well. I will make sure of that.

"Hey, Jordan! Wake up, man. Is you asleep?"

My mind must been working overtime because it seems like it was only a second ago that I closed my eyes. Slowly I open my eyes to notice we are directly behind my car. Somehow I must have gotten lost in the root of my thoughts to the point of not noticing how long I had my eyes closed.

"Naw, man, I wasn't asleep at all, just resting my eyes, doing some serious thinking. Thanks for the ride back to my car as well as everything you did for me so far…much respect. Text me the address to the club. I will see you tonight fo' sho'."

With my right foot out the door, Alfonzo grabs my shoulder before I could make it fully out his ride. Watching him turn the radio down a li'l lower as he was about to speak, I stare at him in mystery of what else he had to say.

"I know you have a lot on your mind, but just know this, man… everything will work out in God's time. Like my grandma would say all the time, it may not happen when you wanted it, but it will always come on time. Whatever your dreams are, it will come true."

"I hear ya, man, thanks."

I watch Alfonzo pull off as he enters the busy streets of downtown Detroit. There's nothing I want more than to finally have a face-to-face talk with my girl. Even though we're taking a break, she's still my girl within. In time she will find herself right back with me. We're having a few differences that are leading to a minor setback, but we'll get over it. The last conversation we had was simply volatile, but I'm happy it happened because it woke my ass up. Now that I'm awake, I can have a heart-to-heart conversation with my girl. If I take the long way to Destiny's crib, it will give me some more time to get my thoughts together. Also I think calling my right-hand man, for a li'l bit of advice will be something I can use. Placing the phone in my hand before taking off into the streets of downtown Detroit, my phone starts to ring. This time I made sure it was someone I wanted to talk to before answering. Oh boy, it's my uncle. I know he's going to say shit to make me laugh.

"Hello, Unk."

"Hey, nephew, how you been?"

"I'm okay, and you?"

"I'm good. Beverly and I about to go to grocery store to pick up a few groceries for the cookout lata on. We all miss ya. When you coming back to visit?"

"I'm not sure, Unk. It's possible that it will be sooner than you think. Destiny and I are taking a break."

"Awww! So that's what got you sounding like a whiny girl over the phone. I can tell in your voice something's on your mind. I've known you before you had the courage to even talk to a female. The way you sounding, I already knew it was about a woman."

My uncle's right; I should've just told him that I'm not okay instead of trying to hide it. He was the one who educated me on the topic of sex. My mama tried to but failed in my opinion. The more she would tell me to wait until I get married, the more I wanted to experiment with the female body and the more I would fantasize about women in sweet wet dreams. My uncle on the other hand would tell me whenever I decide to have sex to make sure I used protection, because he don't see me with no nappy-headed babies running around here. He would even give me advice on how to get girls to sleep with me. He would school me on how to sweet-talk a girl enough to get her panties so wet that she wouldn't refuse having sex with me. This will be my first time coming to him about a relationship issue since this is the first relationship I tried to take seriously.

"After I received some of the best news in my life about getting approved for a business loan, I cooked and prepared an evening for the both of us. In my mind, cooking and running her a hot bubble bath after work was showing how much I appreciate her for introducing me to someone who could help get my business started. In return, she told me that she wants space…that we need time apart."

"Oh, so she hit with the need-space line. I'm surprised she didn't say, 'It's not you, it's me.'"

"She couldn't say that classic bullshit line because it's not her, it's me. I fucked up."

"What you do?"

"In simple terms, I allowed my emotions dealing with Samuel cloud my way of thinking. I worked so hard trying to prove to myself and everyone that I'm nothing like him. I wanted Destiny to bear my child so I could prove that I'm a better dad than he ever could be. I know it sounds stupid."

"Naw, Jay, it doesn't sound stupid. I know you don't like your dad. Hell, I don't like his punk ass much, but my sister loves him. Since my sister loves him, I will respect that. She's a grown woman, and I refuse to make a decision for her as long as he doesn't lay a hand on her. I won't kick his ass. I do think that you're being a li'l selfish with your decision making. You want a kid to prove to another man you better than him. When raising a child, you should do it because you ready to, not because you trying to prove that you better than someone."

"You're right."

"You know I have nothing but tough love for ya. I can't allow my nephew to be soft."

I love talking to my uncle because he always knows how to lighten the mood with his humor. Everything he says to me always seems to be so influencing that I can't disagree. Before having a highly sentimental talk with Destiny, I need a li'l humor.

"Well, Unk, I'm pulling up at Destiny's place now, so I will talk to you lata."

"Okay, you make sure you make things right with her because out all the other hoes you shown me, I can tell you care about this young lady. Take care, and I will check on you lata."

"Okay, Unk, will do."

As I slowly get out my car after turning the ignition off, I take a deep breath then exhale. This is going to be more difficult than anything I ever experienced before. I'm an emotional wreck. In all my twenty-two years, I have never seek as much advice that I have over the last couple of days. Not only have I been seeking advice from multiple people, I'm about to reveal mental scars that I never wanted to show anyone. I know she's here because her car is parked outside, so it's time to man up.

Each step I take closer to her apartment door makes my shoes feel as if there's wet cement on them. I'm facing the inevitable. At some point in my life, I had to start owning up to the issues I have with Samuel. After revealing to her why I pushed so hard for a child, she will understand. She will soon see how quick I've grown in such a short period of time. I'm a man now, not a boy.

I knock timidly at the door, waiting for her to open up. At this point, I'm not sure what she would say. I'm not sure what I would say since my thoughts are all over the place. I raise my fist toward the door to knock again, but before I could, she opens the door wide. Her hair pulled back, with no makeup on, she's standing in the door with some tights and a tank top on. I always thought she looks absolutely stunning with no makeup on. Natural beauty will always prevail over artificial enhancement.

"Come in," Destiny says in a soft whisper as she steps aside, inviting me in.

Walking past her, I smell her peculiar scent of the two perfumes she likes to mix together. It only reminds me of how much I love being around her. I sit down on the sofa as she closes the door, making her way toward me. Now that she sits close to me, I feel comfortable again, unlike how I felt walking to the front door.

"I stopped by to finally sit down and have a rational conversation. I'm not happy with how things went down the last time I was here."

"Neither did I. The timing of exposing how I felt about our relationship was awful. After spending all that time preparing something special for me, I could've waited to drop something like that on you. I do apologize."

"You know, I don't think…well, I know I haven't been totally honest with you. Countless times you asked me why I insist on having children, so soon. I would always ignore the question. Now I'm ready to have that talk."

"Okay, I'm listening," Destiny says with a deep sigh.

"As you already know, Samuel and I don't have the best father-and-son relationship, which leads to the internal reconstruction I'm going through today. My whole life I've been afraid to let go of the negative energy I've been having inside of me toward Samuel. What will happen if I do forgive him and work on repairing our bond? If I forgive him, he probably just find a way to fuck it up. Last night, an epiphany came to me that I need to let the negative energy go. Perhaps the situation between Samuel and me can be resolved if I learn to forgive. Once I start to work towards forgiving him, hopefully my burden of trying to be better than him will go away."

"I understand, baby. I never knew you felt like this. Trust me, no one, including me, doesn't think you will make the same mistakes as your father. I know you better than that. I think you should forgive him. In time you will know if there's a chance of repairing the father-and-son relationship."

"I think I'm ready to take that risk now. My family back home told me that Samuel and my mama been happier than ever. I guess he really has changed. If we can build a strong father-and-son bond, then I want to carry the burden of trying to be a better father than him in the future."

A tear sails down Destiny's face as she starts to become emotional listening to me speak. I imagine she is crying because she's never seen this side of me. She probably didn't expect for us to have a conversation like this. Looking at her cry is flabbergasting because I only seen the stronger side of her. All these years of knowing her, along with the arguments, I never seen her shed one tear until now. I'm already heavy with various emotions, and seeing her cry didn't help. I feel myself sinking in a flood of my own feelings, trying desperately to hold my head above water. My energy is low, causing my legs and arms to get tired. The flood of water has overpowered me as I pull Destiny near, kissing her tear away as we both cry together.

"Destiny, don't cry, babe."

"I understand now why you want children. You wanted to prove to yourself that you can be a better father than Samuel. I think you will be a wonderful dad, but I'm just not ready for a family."

"I realize I'm not ready either."

With our forehead touching, lips less than an inch apart, I got lost in the moment. I wipe a tear away with my thumb as I hold the side of her face with my hands before touching her lips with mine. The more we kiss, the more aggressive she starts to be. She rips away at my T-shirt like it were a piece of paper, pushes me back on the sofa as she jumps on top of me. We continue licking and biting on each other's lips as

I rip her tank top off exposing her erotic chocolate-shape milk buds, ready for them to melt in my mouth. Instantly I feel the moisture of her crouch against mine. As my tongue dances around her nipple, she holds my head in her arms while moaning. I listen to her sing the most beautiful song I heard in my life. She sounds sweeter than a southern hummingbird in the middle of the summer.

Once I pick her up off the sofa, I continue to lick on her body as she locks her legs around my waist. With all my concentration on her, I lay her down on the soft on her back. I lick my way down to her belly ring, occasionally kissing her in the process of making my way down to taste her wetness. One glance at her face as I work my way down, I witness her eyes close as her mouth opens like she was thirsty for more. With my mouth and hands, I pull down her tights while she rises up enough for me to pull them down. Without hesitation, I start tonguing her other lips as this was going to be my last supper. Minutes go by before her legs started shaking as she reaches her first climax. Her breathing had increased as I was more than ready to get inside of her.

Without an intermission, I pull down my B-ball shorts and boxers so that I can ease up inside of her. With her legs clutched around me, I start to go faster deeper inside the rainstorm. The warmth of the storm, along with the wetness of it all, is so pleasurable that I am in a trance. Never came over here with the intentions to break down crying like a wimp, but now after we cried together, we made love. The fact that I'm massaging the most inner muscle of her as I caress every part of her body, I can say shedding a few tears was all worth it. This what the O'Jays was talking about when they made the hit "Cry Together." Growing up I would hear the song a lot at home. My mama would play this song on repeat, especially after she was making up with Samuel. What I'm feeling right now I can feel this way for the rest of my life.

I had the best sex I experienced in my life, or what I should call as my first passionate lovemaking experience. Don't get me wrong; all the other times we had sex, I loved my woman, but this time, it seems different. It feels like we connect on a deeper level since I let my guard down. We lie together butt naked on the sofa as I my head rests on her chest, drifting asleep as I lie and rest.

BREAK UP TO MAKE UP

I imagine hours went by before I woke up alone on the sofa with a blanket over my naked body. I'm not surprised that Destiny manages to sneak away from me while I fell asleep on her chest. It's not that she's sneaky; I'm just not a light sleeper. The only thing that can wake me up from a good rest is the smell of food. That's just what woke me up once again as I sniff the air, indulging in the smell of what seems to be pizza. Whatever kind of pizza it is, I hope it came from Papa John's. Destiny knows that's my favorite fast-food pizza restaurant. Gathering my B-ball shorts while glancing at the clock, I notice that it's well over in the evening. I imagine she ordered pizza for the two of us. With my nose open wide, I walk into the kitchen as she sets the table with a bowl of salad, a glass of wine, and some plates to place our food. She looks up at me with a smile.

"I knew the smell of food would wake you."

"Somehow it always does. You know me like a book."

"Yes, I know you pretty well, huh?"

I playfully dance my way over to her as I lean toward her to place a kiss on her lips. Together we giggle. Somehow we work our way back on good terms. It's amazing how we're in the same space making each other laugh again. I'm enjoying our time together.

"Someone has two left feet."

"So you got jokes. You know you love my dance moves."

"Right," she says with a light chuckle. "Now let's sit down and eat. We have some more things to discuss."

"Yes, let's eat because I'm starving. What else do you want to talk about?"

"I want to discuss the status of our relationship."

"I agree that's something we need to touch base on."

Now that I sit across the table in front of her, all I could think about is how I want us to get back together. After she finished saying a prayer over the food, I'm going plead my case how we should pick up where we left off. We're in a good place right now. Our communication is better than it has ever been.

"I want to thank you for opening your heart to me and allowing me inside your world. I feel as if I learned more about the way you think in a few minutes than I have since we been dating. I couldn't imagine how it feels to battle with mental distress that divided household has put on you throughout your childhood. Imagine if one of my parents was in and out of my life growing up, I would be a mess."

"I realize I have to take it a day at a time when working on forgiving him. However, I still want to work on us in the meantime. Unlike before, I won't allow my unresolved issues with Samuel come between us. I've decided that I'm going to move back to Atlanta and work on rebuilding a relationship with both of my parents."

"Jay, I think that's a wonderful idea. Now that we our stabilizing our relationship more on communication, I believe that we can work on us. Perhaps we can work on starting over instead of picking up where we left off. You know, just laughing, talking, and supporting each other like we did when we first started dating. I know the distance will be a factor again, but we can make it work."

"I will like to start over. This time we will make time to see each other more often regardless of the distance," I say as I felt her foot resting in my lap.

She always likes resting her foot in my lap at home while we sit across the dining table eating our meal. She also knows her petite foot massaging my manhood would turn me on. We both know that it would only lead to one thing. Usually she would only tease me like that when she wants me to take charge after we finished eating.

"When you plan on moving back?"

"I'm going talk to Markus about letting me stay with him for a while until I find my own place. As soon as next week, I plan on moving back if possible. I will drive."

"Let me know when you going so I can take time off work and meet you down there. I will be there to support you. Plus we can spend time with Markus and Asia like we used to back in college. It would be fun."

"Okay, will do."

After dinner, we indulge in more heavenly minutes of passionate lovemaking. We paint images of our body through sound with a thousand and one *ohhhs* and *awwws*. The rhythms of our body crashing together are smoother than the waves rushing onto the ocean's shore. Our breathing increases as moisture flows down every angle of our down as we continue to show a blueprint for the love we have for each other.

CLUB LIBERAL

Hours went by before I woke up on the floor in the bedroom from round 2 of lovemaking. This girl got that comeback "put you to sleep kind" of love. I simply can't get enough. As it gets closer to dark, I try to convince Destiny to come along with me to pick up the rest of my valuables that I left at Alfonzo's, but she says she's tired and wants to stay at home. When her mind is made up, there's no changing it. If I wasn't so curious about why I was supposed to leave a close mind at the door, I wouldn't go to Alfonzo and Byron's club tonight. The curiosity of why they look at it as the most prestigious business investment that was ever made keeps my interest. On second thought, I suppose everyone feels that way about something or someone they're investing in.

Tonight I want to be comfortable as well as casual. There's no dress code, so I'm just going to wear some blue cargo shorts with some Nike Jordan's and a white collared Polo shirt. On the way back to Novi, Markus and I can probably talk on the phone. Markus will be proud to hear my plans of coming home. He's been carrying most of the workload for getting our sports bar up and running for a while now. Like my uncle said, I've been kind of selfish. I haven't been thinking about how slack I've been on being a co-owner. Markus has been setting up business meeting with building contractors and lawyers and discussing getting our liquor licenses from the state of Georgia while I been pouting about bullshit that I shouldn't even be thinking about at the moment.

The phone rings only about two times before Markus answered. He must damn near be right next to his phone or expecting a call. I wasn't expecting him to answer so soon.

"What up, Jay?"

"Nothing much, about to head out for a party Alfonzo invited me to at his club. What you up to?"

"Asia and I at Stone Mountain Park about to watch some fireworks."

"I have some good news."

"What is it?"

"I'm moving back to Atlanta. I need one favor though. Will it be okay with you and Asia if I stay in your guest room until I find my own spot?"

"Of course, you can stay. I know Asia well enough to know that she won't mind helping out a friend. Why the sudden move? Is everything okay between you and Destiny?"

"We broke up for a brief moment but now working on starting over. Actually, after I learned how to express my feelings as opposed to holding back so much, our connection is growing strong. Now we back to just having fun along with enjoying each other's company."

"That's good. I'm happy for the both of you. When you plan on coming back?"

"Next week. I'm just going tell my job that I have to move back because of a family emergency."

"I'm happy to know you coming back."

"I plan on having that long delayed chat with my parents. The talk with Samuel is long overdue."

"Wow. I can see someone ready to forgive. If you need any support, I got your back. You're like my brother."

"I know you got my back, you always have since I'd known you. Plus it's time for me to pull my weight with getting our sports bar up and running."

"True. Let me get back to Asia, because she got some of her nieces and nephews with us. They bad as hell. I don't know why she agreed to her family members to take them with us. It's a reason why they were trying to get rid of them."

"All right, man. I will see ya soon. And make sure you don't strangle one or all the kids."

"I may just have to choke one of them, so keep ya eye on the news," Markus says with a hint of humor in his voice. "A'ight, man, see ya soon."

It didn't take me no time to get to Club Liberal. Once Alfonzo texted me the address, I placed the info in my GPS, and it got me here in no time. From the outside the club looks spacious, also very conspicuous with how the letters of the club blink one at a time in rotation. After all the lights blink at once, they all blink at the same time for about a minute. The lights are red, white, and blue. Seem as if someone had a vision for not just the name but the theme of how they wanted the club to look as well. Based on the line outside, it must be the place to be as I witness a variety of people in the line. Good thing I'm on the guest list because I'm not in the mood to wait in a long-ass line.

Walking my way up to the club, it looks like I see Destiny's neighbor in line with his boyfriend. After taking a double look, it is official. That's his gay ass in the line with his arched eyebrows, two sizes too small jeans with a shirt on that barely covers his bellybutton. He's so over the top. I never could understand how he could go out the house comfortably dressed like that. Like always, I never speak and never stare, just act like he's invisible. Out of all the clubs in the state of Michigan, why the hell he want to be at a straight club?

"I'm Jordan Rodgers. My name should be on the guest list," I say to one of the bouncers.

"Yes. I see it come on through. Enjoy your night."

That's weird; he didn't pat me down. I guess, since I'm on the guest list, Alfonzo and Byron don't instruct the security to pat guests down, or maybe they know I'm not going come in here with a weapon on me. Whatever, I'm in this bitch now, so I'm just going buy me a drink and make sure I have a good time.

The first thing I notice was, the color scheme matches the same color scheme as the flashing lights outside. My guess is the colors supposed to represent freedom of speech or expression. In many ways, it all makes sense to me. The good old USA does preach equal rights in its constitution, so to go with the American color scheme for a club name after the word *liberal* makes tons of sense. The club set is remarkable that I barely pay attention to the crowd. Each booth has its own theme. One booth has a stripper pole, while one booth has more cowboy theme with a mechanic bull in the middle of the booth. The booth

I love the most is the sports setting with a pool table and air hockey table. I'm sure every penny spent on each booth in here is worth it.

Now that I'm by the bar with my drink, I stop admiring the club to notice everyone around me. The crowd is not only diverse when it comes to ethnic background but with sexual preferences as well. I look to my left and see a stud, or what we all know as a woman who carries herself as a man, dancing with a woman. Why in the world would a woman be twerking on another woman? I mean, it ain't like she's going feel nothing but her jeans against her ass. Most men think it's sexy; I think it's silly. I look straight ahead; now I see two men dancing with the same chick while looking at each other with lust in their eyes. What in the hell is going on in this club? I'm not longer mesmerized by the layout or the booths. The people here and their actions are starting to make me feel uncomfortable; if I continue to see bizarre behavior, I'm leaving.

Taking my shot of Parton to the head, I turn to the right of me, only to witness Alfonzo and Byron on the dance floor, bumping and grinding all over each other. What the fuck going on here? This is why they didn't know how to explain why I should leave a closed mind at the door. Never did I say I would or wouldn't be open-minded, but this is damn right despicable to see another brother, or any man for that matter, on another man like that. With pure disbelief all over my face, I start to walk out the club. Making my way through the crowd, I am ready to punch someone in their shit if they touch or look at me the wrong way.

Out the corner of my eye, I see Alfonzo approaching me. Shit. I didn't think he saw me running toward the exit since he was so engaged in dancing with Byron. If he catches up with me, I may just ask him why he didn't give me a better heads-up about his club. I didn't come here for this. Matter of fact, I think he owes me an explanation, so I will stick around long enough for that. Almost near the exit, I turn around as Alfonzo is almost at arm's reach of me. I can't hear him speak over the loud music, but reading his lips, I can see that he's calling my name. Seconds later he stood in front of me with a confused look.

"Yo, Jordan, I didn't know you was here. You were going leave without speaking?"

"Hell yeah! You didn't tell me this is a gay club or that you and Bryon fucking around."

His body language tells me he got somewhat offended while his facial expression showed humiliation, like I did something wrong to him. He's the one who led me to an awful event without notification if I would be comfortable. If he wants to turn up in this bitch, we can. I won't back down, or we can go outside so I can stomp him in the streets. I never was afraid to fight when I have to.

"Let's go outside so we can talk. It's too noisy in here."

"After you."

Never will I turn my back on him, especially now because if he wants to fight, I don't want him behind me. I need to see what he's doing at all time. He might be one of them dirty type of dudes who like to fight unfair. Once we got outside, I tell him where I parked, giving him directions as I walk beside him with my fist balled tight, ready to swing if he tried something I didn't like.

"Okay, we made it to my car…so talk."

"Bryon and I didn't tell you about us because what we do in our spare time is our business. We don't owe an explanation to anyone including you about if or how we fucking around. However, I do apologize for the both of us for not telling you that our club allows gay men and women in our establishment. No, this club isn't just for gay people. We allow anyone to come out to have a good time. You only saw what you wanted to see. There are heterosexual couples in there. Not everyone is closed minded when it comes to their sexuality as you."

"I should've known that you and Byron messing around. Oh, boy knows his way around the kitchen like he cooks for you all the time. He even got up and started washing the dishes like he's your bitch."

"Hold up. I won't allow you to disrespect him like that. Don't forget we allowed you to come into our home when you were in need. Now you may not like our relationship, but you will respect it."

"This conversation is over. I'm done," I say as I open my door to get in my car.

"Remember, gay men aren't the only ones carrying their feelings on the down low. There's many men who hide who they are in the dark because they afraid of what others may think of them. You of all people should know."

Without allowing him to preach another word, I spun off, burning rubber as I left the parking spot. How could I carry on a friendship with him knowing that he likes men? In his mind he could be plotting on making a move on me. I'm a man, so I do know how men think. Men can have someone special in our life but still fantasize about someone else from time to time. A man can claim a chick his best friend, but in the back of his mind he's scheming on how he going get that. No one can explain why men think about sex so much or are visual creatures. That's why men don't allow their women to be around a bunch of male friends without him being around even if they're mutual friends. Most men find it hard to trust another man around his woman when he's not around.

With that being said in this scenario, I don't want to be the guy that Alfonzo visualize naked. Then again, I probably can trust that Alfonzo wouldn't cross that line. He never did anything wrong to me. In fact, as long as he's been in my life as friend, he has opened my eyes to see that I need to shed light on a few issues that no one else could make me see even if they shed light on it for me. In all my years of knowing that there're homosexual individuals in the world, I never imagine befriending any of them. As of now, maybe it's possible. I owe that to Alfonzo for opening my eyes that not every gay man wants or tries to fit the stereotype I had in mind. One thing I am sure about is I would hate to lose a good homeboy over something that doesn't have anything to do with me. How Alfonzo and Byron choose to live their life is their prerogative.

MOVING FORWARD

After about what seem like endless hours of driving from Detroit, Michigan, to Social Circle, Georgia, I feel exhausted. My ass is tired from sitting down for so long as well as my right leg's been catching cramps from driving an extended period of time. I drove straight here nonstop. It wouldn't be a bad idea to stop by Markus's crib to put away some of my things as well as get some rest. Since I been on the road, I've been anxiously waiting to meet my parents for that much-delayed talk. With nerves riding high, I only made stops to fill up on gas during my long journey. Surprisingly, my mama hasn't noticed I'm out here in her driveway yet as I wait for Destiny to meet up with me. I'm not afraid to admit I need her support.

The last few months have been full of surprises that I will never forget. Out of everything that has happened over the past months, I believe everything happens for a reason. For every experience, no matter how awkward it was, I can honestly say every obstacle has molded me into a better man. No longer do I have the same mind frame as I used to have. I'm breaking out…braking free from the shell that I allowed society to put me in. As I sit here today with my windows down listening to Mary J. Blige, I can honestly say I don't give a shit who hears me listening to R&B music alone. Listening to R&B music alone doesn't make me soft. I believe the ones who are truly soft are the ones who follow the crowd. Anytime you do something to cover up who you really are because you're afraid of what someone will think of you, the punk is really you. A strong individual who stands on his own two feet without the opinion of others to undergird his or her beliefs is the ruler of his or her sentiments. From this day and beyond I, want to be a ruler while I'm regnant over my beliefs.

Alfonzo taught me that covering up what bothers you along with pretending that everything is fine do not make you masculine. Just because you hide the truth in the dark doesn't mean that it won't rip you apart. At some point, what you try to keep locked away will break out and expose the truth. The day I found out he's gay broke down all typical thoughts I had about gay men. I always thought I could notice a gay man because I didn't think they can hide their flamboyances, sort of like Destiny's neighbor. Not all gay men are loud and in your face with their sexuality. There're men out there who don't arch their eyebrows, twist their hips, or refer to themselves as Queen Bee.

The guys who try so desperately to fit in with whom they think are their homeboys should know they're not that different from the fellas on the down low. Straight fellas and DL men have more in common than they know, because just like the fellas on the down low, they desperately want to fit in. I'm a straight man. Now I can honestly say I don't have that in common with the men on the low because I'm freeing myself from all barriers. I'm going do what's best for me to grow as a man, not what I think others want me to be.

Looking in my rearview mirror, I notice Destiny pulling up in her rental car, pulling up in a black Mercedes, which doesn't have me appalled because she likes being flashy. We make eye contact as I continue looking through the rearview. After she took her sunglasses off, I can tell she must be smiling as I see her eyes sparkle as she smiles. I watch in awe as she gets out the car, looking exquisite with accessories around her neck and wrist. Her hair is pulled back to draw more attention to her stunning face. My baby is fitting that sundress perfectly.

"Sorry I'm a few minutes late. It took forever to finally get my rental car. They claim because they was back up with a lot of clients renting cars."

"It's okay. No one has been out here yet, so the both of them must be so occupied that they didn't notice I'm out here."

"Well, get out the car, sweetie. I know you nervous, but everything will be fine."

This is the moment I drove all this way for. There's no time to turn around now. At this very moment, I seem to be chopped and screwed…in other words, while the situation seems to be moving at a fast pace, I seem to be moving at a slow pace. I just need to relax. Destiny opens the car door, pulls me by the hand until I got out, and then kisses me softly on the lips.

"You will be fine," she whispers in my ear.

"Thanks for showing up…it means a lot."

Feeling more vibrant knowing that I got such stable support system within my Destiny, I'm more than ready to work on the shattered relationship I have with my parents. We make our way toward the door, I could hear the O'Jays playing "Cry Together," so this could mean that they must have had an argument and in the works of making up. I swear if he hurt my mama again, I will beat his ass. With rage in my eyes, I knock on the door as if I'm the feds with a search warrant. What seems like two seconds, I hear footsteps approaching at a swift pace. With panic in her voice, my mama yells out, "Who is it?"

"Ya, son, open up."

The door swings open fast. Instead of it being my mama, it is Samuel who stood in the doorway with nothing but his pajamas on. I can see my mama behind him as she uses him as a shield while she fixes her nightgown. I already know what they were up to. This explains why neither one of them noticed me pull up. My mama's hair all wild while sweat running down Samuel's face explains a lot. I guess their marriage is on good terms for good this time.

"Y'all come on in. Is there anything I can get y'all…something to drink or something to eat?" Samuel says as he smiles as he was happy to see me.

"Naw, Dad, I just came to talk and to get reacquainted with my parents."

"I will like that, son," my parents say at the same time.

Even though we both procrastinated for years on rebuilding our father-and-son relationship, now seems like a good place to start.

ABOUT THE AUTHOR

Casempium Q. Johnson is originally from Social Circle, Georgia, but currently resides in the Atlanta, Georgia area. Shortly after earning a bachelor's degree in Information Technology he found his true passion, which is writing. The world can definitely expect more from this talented young writer as he continues to demonstrate his creativity through his stories.

CPSIA information can be obtained
at www.ICGtesting.com
Printed in the USA
LVHW04s0021161018
593746LV00003B/295/P